FATIGUE TO

Vitality

How to win the battle
against cholesterol,
prevent degenerative diseases
and live the
healthiest lifestyle!

**NICHOLAS
DELGADO**

*Author of Weight Loss and Energy Now
and Zero Cholesterol Weight Loss Cookbook*

FATIGUE TO VITALITY

Published in the United States of America
by Delgado Medical
16787 Beach Bl. # 202
Huntington Beach, Calif. 92647

ISBN - 1-879084-02-3

TABLE OF CONTENTS

INTRODUCTION

Nicholas R. Delgado, Jr., is the Founder and Director of the Delgado Health Plan. After graduating from U.S.C. with a degree in Psychology, he began his postgraduate studies in Physical Therapy at U.S.C's Rancho Los Amigos Hospital, followed by volunteer work at Daniel Freeman Hospital and Chino Hospital. Through his experiences in physical therapy, Mr. Delgado became deeply concerned by the large numbers of people dying from such degenerative diseases as atherosclerosis, stroke, diabetes and cancer.

Because of this work, he was motivated to undertake in-depth postgraduate studies in nutrition at Loma Linda University, Cal State Los Angeles and Cal State Long Beach. He also spent hundreds of hours studying medical journals at U.S.C. and U.C. Irvine in his search for solutions to degenerative diseases. He began to apply what he was learning to his medical problems (obesity and high blood pressure). After just 5 months he showed dramatic reductions in his weight (50 lbs.), blood pressure (from 200/90 to 110/70) and cholesterol (from 186 to 118). Eventually Mr. Delgado freed himself of medications.

Mr. Delgado then developed his highly successful nutrition, exercise, motivation and stress management program (forerunner to today's Delgado Health Plan). In 1979, Nick Delgado was asked to become the Director of the Pritikin Better Health Program by the famous research scientist, Nathan Pritikin. Mr. Delgado held that position for three years. During this period he met and studied with many world renowned scientists, including Denis Burkitt, M.D., Ernest Wynder, M.D., and Dr. Cleaves Bennett. In 1982 Mr. Delgado was appointed President of Dr. Fox's Lifestyle program, headquartered in Beverly Hills, California. He then went on to create a dynamic new program, featuring seminars to the public that could be sponsored by medical clinics as a community service.

In December 1982 the Delgado Health Plan began education and medical services in Southern California. Seminars and counseling services were provided by Nick Delgado and Bea Delgado. Since the inception of the Delgado Medical Clinic, our staff of doctors and highly trained professionals have enabled thousands of participants to feel renewed. In all, more than 3,000 seminars have been presented to the public at medical clinics, hospitals, community centers and large corporations including Aerospace and TRW.

This book combines the collective experiences of the Delgado Medical staff in helping people like yourself. Perhaps you have a health problem, or maybe you would like to experience optimum health. Read this book, start exercising, begin the nutrition plan and you can benefit and improve in the following areas:

HEART DISEASE & HARDENING OF THE ARTERIES: Most of the known factors that lead to artery closures will be lowered or eliminated. Your blood cholesterol level may drop an average of 20% (the harmful LDL will come down the most, while the good HDL stabilizes). You can reduce or eliminate medications for heart disease, angina, hypertension, diabetes and obesity with the assistance of our team of medical doctors.

ARTHRITIS: As you learn to improve your circulation, you can reduce the pain and stiffness in your joints.

ANEMIA: It is important to identify the cause of your blood's reduced ability to carry oxygen first, and then find a solution that is best for you. We have found the Delgado Health Plan of nutrition and exercise can build up the deficient blood. Your need may include iron, B-12, folic acid, Vitamin E and Vitamin C, which can all be found in whole natural foods.

Sometimes allergies to foods like dairy products can cause a severe case of iron deficiency, which is well documented in medical literature.

ASTHMA & EMPHYSEMA: As your lung capacity improves through our program of mild aerobic exercises, improved nutrition to reduce fatty blood, and smoking cessation assistance (if needed), you can experience enhanced breathing capabilities.

CANCER: The National Cancer Institute and the American Cancer Society now fully support the contention that cancer is in large part preventable, and even if it should develop, there is new evidence to show that cancer of the breast, prostate, colon and uterus is treatable. Research on a low-fat, zero cholesterol, high-fiber diet (the Delgado-type plan) has shown exciting results in the fight against cancer.

CONSTIPATION, HEMORRHOIDS, COLITIS, DIVERTICULOSIS, ULCERS, VARICOSE VEINS AND GALLSTONES: These digestive disorders can be prevented, or, if present, often relieved by following the Delgado Program because of the use of natural fibers and exercise to stimulate and properly soothe the digestive tract.

PROSTATE DISORDERS, MALE SEXUAL IMPOTENCE: Can be helped through proper medical management using various solutions based on your specific needs. An alarming number of men develop prostate cancer. Evidence shows that cases could be prevented by maintaining a low cholesterol level. Avoiding the accumulation of cholesterol is of critical importance to the health of the prostate gland. A high cholesterol level is now considered a leading cause of sexual impotence due to clogged arteries and restricted blood flow to the penis.

HIGH BLOOD PRESSURE (HYPERTENSION): By following the six effective steps to controlling blood pressure as outlined in this plan, you may free yourself of the need for medications in just twelve weeks.

KIDNEY & LIVER DISORDERS: A high protein diet, alcohol and fat inhibit the function and damage these vital organs. The Delgado Plan offers accepted solutions.

DIABETES, HYPOGLYCEMIA: The Delgado Program has generated considerable excitement within the medical community through its success in helping people to reach their ideal blood sugar levels in as little as eight weeks using the high complex carbohydrate diet. This type of plan is now being recommended by the American Diabetic Association.

GLAUCOMA, CATARACTS: There are people in the world who rarely develop these eye disorders so common in our culture. Medical research shows that excess fat in the bloodstream can lead to a pressure buildup in the eye, damaging the retina (nerves in the eye) that can cause the progressive loss of eyesight. The Delgado Plan can reduce the interocular pressure in the eye and prevent the need for eye drops. Many cases of cataracts are related to high cholesterol levels, eye drops for glaucoma and impurities (sorbitol), which ruin the clarity of the lens. You can look forward to a life virtually free of these eye disorders by following our program.

MENSTRUAL DISORDERS (PMS), MENOPAUSE: The use of the Delgado Program for female hormone imbalances is safe and effective without the need for drugs. Daily exercise and a low-fat diet are the cornerstone therapys that are safer than hormone replacement drugs.

OSTEOPOROSIS: By following our simple guidelines, exercises and recipes you can prevent and restore the loss of bone material.

OBESITY, WEIGHT LOSS OR GAIN, IDEAL WEIGHT: Finally, by following a simple program of improved nutrition and exercise you can reduce the size of your fat cells to ideal level. The result: you attain your ideal weight!

The Delgado Medical staff would like you to live a longer, healthier, happier life. Living a longer, healthier life is important to you and your family, isn't it? And yet, there is a myth about life expectancy in the United States. Because of our lower infant mortality rate, people mistakenly think we're healthier; however, past the age of 40, we rank 38th in the world in life expectancy in a recent study comparing 60 nations! Though our country has the best of medical technology, you still have a greater chance than ever before of dying prematurely from atherosclerosis, heart disease, cancer, diabetes or hypertension. In fact, 1 1/2 million people die every year from these causes alone.

If you were to drop dead suddenly from heart disease without any debilitating symptoms, that might not be so bad. But it doesn't usually work that way. Most people in their last 20 years of life slowly lose functions - hearing, sight, etc. Their joints ache, blood pressure rises, there are side effects from medications, sexual impotency occurs and they lose their zest for life. If you could discover how to reduce or prevent these and other serious illnesses - how to achieve the ideal level of health, and significantly extend your life - you would, wouldn't you? The Delgado Medical Program is now available to you as a complete educational, motivational and personalized approach. It can help you and your family to improve the quality of life.

Comparing your health to people in optimum or ideal health provides helpful insight. There are over 800 million people on the Delgado Health Plan type of diet: high in complex carbohydrates and fiber, low in fat and cholesterol. In these countries (25 populations examined) we find almost no killer diseases such as heart disease, and they have a longer life expectancy past the age of 40. In contrast, one out of every three adults in this country is suffering from cardiovascular disease. What is wrong with the American diet? Could it be that the fast foods, TV dinners and high levels of sugar, fat, cholesterol and salt that we were raised on lead to illness and heart disease? Combine these with a lack of exercise, obesity or smoking and your risk for developing heart disease climbs even higher.

Heart disease is gradual. The average closure of the 20-year-old's coronary arteries is already 20%. The average closure of a 35-year-old is almost 50%. When you are 45 years of age, you may have a 90% closure and it's at this late stage that you'll have your first symptom: angina (chest pain). If your arteries to the brain narrow, you may have signs of dizziness, headaches, senility or even stroke.

The tragedy is that most people with so-called "average" cholesterol levels of 160 to 280 have hardening (narrowing) of the arteries. If you're smart, you'll want to prevent further damage to your arteries. The Delgado Plan can help you do this by bringing your cholesterol level down to safer levels. Dr. W. Castelli, cardiologist, has stated that "diet could reverse (dissolve) coronary artery disease plaques in 90% of the patients if we got everyone's cholesterol below 150 mg."

Following heart disease, cancer is the second major cause of death in the U.S. If you could learn sensible guidelines to prevent 50-80% of the cases of cancer (specifically breast, prostate and colon), you would follow them wouldn't you? In this book, we explain a dramatic nutrition program, which according to the National Cancer Institute and the American Cancer Society is the effective defense against cancer.

The Delgado Plan has also helped people with hypertension to lower their blood pressure to normal, free of medications. This book explains the six effective steps to blood pressure reduction. Without our comprehensive system, most people fail because they usually just reduce salt and use medications. By contrast, we teach you the steps to reducing fat in your circulation that frees your body of stress.

The American Diabetic Association has also found that a Delgado-type approach can successfully help most diabetics to reduce their need for insulin dramatically. According to Dr. Kelly West, endocrinologist, and Dr. James Anderson, 62% of adult onset diabetics could get off insulin and other drugs, and return to ideal health in less than three months.

Like most people, you probably don't have the endurance capabilities of the famous Tarahumara Indians in Northern Mexico, who run nonstop for 48 hours - a distance of 175 miles! They are free of degenerative diseases because they eat a healthy diet and exercise regularly. Their blood relatives, though, the Pima Indians in Phoenix, eat a high fat diet, and as a result have a very high rate of arthritis, diabetes and gallstones.

Is your diet high in fat? Do you know that cheddar cheese and peanut butter are 71% fat? Margarine, corn oil and butter 100% fat and sirloin steak is 77% fat? The average American also eats many hidden fats, because processed sugars also turn into fat. This can cause your bloodstream to become clogged with fats, resulting in poor circulation.

We at the Delgado Medical Clinic believe that whole natural foods, low in fat, low in cholesterol, are your best medicine. Exercise, a positive attitude, and a spiritual commitment will provide the most comprehensive known program leading you on the path to good health. We have medical doctors and health educators who are dedicated to helping you achieve your goals following the Delgado Plan.

For more information, or to make an appointment at our clinic, write to our P.O. Box at Delgado Medical 16787 Beach Bl. # 202 Huntington Beach CA 92647 or call us at (800) 540-Nick(6425).

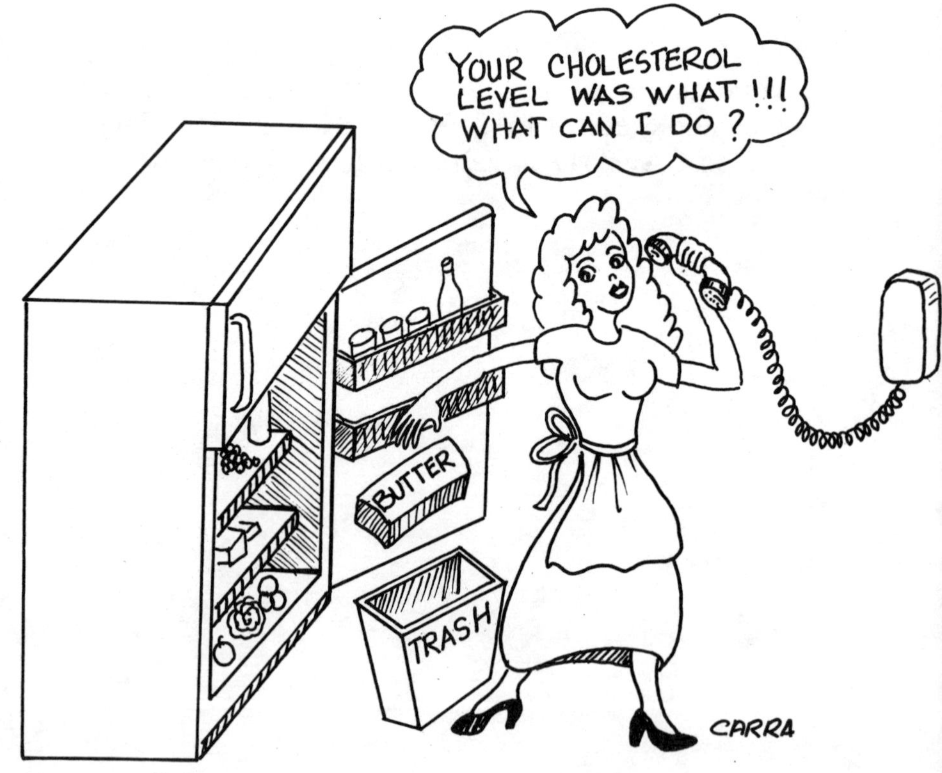
YOUR CHOLESTEROL
LEVEL WAS WHAT !!!
WHAT CAN I DO ?
BUTTER
TRASH
CARRA

CHAPTER ONE
WHAT IS CHOLESTEROL?
WHAT IS FAT?
WHAT LEVEL IS SAFE?

To defeat atherosclerosis, the major killer in the U.S. (50% of premature deaths), you must first understand the most important blood value - cholesterol. You've heard about the good cholesterol (HDL) and the bad cholesterol (LDL). You've even heard some authorities say you don't have to worry about it. However, I would like to share with you some information about cholesterol I think you need to know.

First, cholesterol is a substance made by every cell in your body. A newborn child is born with a cholesterol level of 60. If the child grows up to adulthood and has never eaten any cholesterol bearing foods (animal based foods), the cholesterol level will never exceed 100 to 120 mg. per every 3 1/2 ounces of blood. In populations where artery closure and heart disease are unknown, adults do not have cholesterol levels above 160 - that figure would be maximum. Usually they have cholesterol levels around 130 to 140. It doesn't make any difference how old they are; it never goes above that level. A study in Texas on 1,490 children (5th to 9th graders) showed a shocking 36%, or 403, of the students already had a cholesterol level more than 180 mg/dl.

That level increases the risk of fatal heart attack by 17% or more, as compared to a safe cholesterol reading of under 160.

Cleveland Clinic reported a case of 17 year old boy with a cholesterol level of 186. This boy experienced some slight chest pain, so the doctors did an EKG that was abnormal. Next, an angiogram (X-ray photography of arteries enhanced by injected dye) of his heart showed a complete blockage of the middle coronary artery. The only reason he was still alive was because colateral circulation (new little blood vessels) had developed enough to feed the heart. If this boy eats like most Americans, he'll continue to eat a breakfast of bacon and eggs, with butter on his toast. He'll have a lunch of cheeseburgers and milkshakes, and a dinner of Kentucky Fried Chicken (egg yolk batter) with gravy (animal fat). With this typical American diet, it is very likely he will become a tragic statistic. His death certificate will read "premature death from coronary heart disease."

In populations with adult cholesterol levels above 160, we find the arteries have started to close. When we study populations with adult cholesterol levels of 180 to 200, probably 20% have serious artery closure. Populations with levels around 200 to 240 have 100% artery closure. In our country the average cholesterol level is about 235 to 240. Autopsy studies on 20-year olds who were accidently killed, showed every individual already had substantial artery closure.

These closures in your arteries are made of cholesterol. The artery closes when boil-like abscesses, which we call plaques, grow inside your artery. If you cut these plaques and analyze them, 84% of the weight is cholesterol and, at later stages, calcium.

At Delgado Medical we are often asked, "What is the difference between fat and cholesterol?" Fat provides calories; yet, in excess it is the major contributor to obesity and to many diseases that affects our culture. A high fat diet of oils, margarine, whole milk, cheese, meat, etc. can increase the levels of fat in your blood (triglycerides) which leads to the risk of:

1. HIGH BLOOD PRESSURE (blood thickened by fat)

2. ARTHRITIS (low oxygen from fat causing destruction of joints)

3. DIABETES (fat desensitizing insulin causing poor glucose control)

4. BREAST AND COLON CANCER (fat causing excessive production of cancer causing hormones and chemicals)

5. CHRONIC FATIGUE (high fat levels in the blood that reduces the oxygen carrying capacity of red blood cells to the brain)

6. GLAUCOMA (fat increases cortisone levels in the eyes causing swelling, restriction of fluid flow that can result in damage to the retinal nerves of the eye and blindness)

7. MULTIPLE SCLEROSIS (fat damages the nerves of the body from reduced oxygen carrying capacity of the blood)

8. ATHEROSCLEROSIS (low oxygen levels caused by fat forces more cholesterol deposits into the arteries)

In comparison, cholesterol is much different from fat. First because cholesterol cannot cause you to gain weight since it lacks calories. Unlike fat, you can't see cholesterol in food, since it's permeated equally throughout all animal tissue. This is why there is just as much cholesterol in the white part of chicken or fish as there is in the skin or fat portions. High cholesterol levels can lead to:

1. ATHEROSCLEROSIS or narrowing of arteries and capillaries.

2. HEART ATTACK from cholesterol blocked arteries to the heart.

3. STROKE (clogged and weakened arteries to the brain).

4. SENILITY (loss of brain function due to clogged arteries).

5. IMPOTENCY (loss of male sexual function due to cholesterol clogging arteries to the penis).

6. PROSTATE CANCER (cholesterol build up in the prostate gland restricts oxygen to the gland inducing mutated cancerous cells).

7. CATARACTS (lens of the eye fills with cholesterol causing blindness).

8. GANGRENE (restricted blood flow to the extremities: fingers, toes, hands and feet, leading to numbness, tissue death and amputation caused by cholesterol build up).

9. KIDNEY FAILURE (clogged arteries to the kidneys).

WHAT IS CHOLESTEROL?

Cholesterol is a substance known as a steroid, and is made by the body for definite purposes. For example, small amounts of cholesterol are needed to produce all sex hormones (estrogen, testosterone, etc.) in the body. Cholesterol is part of nerve cells, and Vitamin D is made by the ultraviolet light from sunshine reacting with a cholesterol layer under the skin called dehydro-cholesterol.

Since cholesterol is not a fat and it provides no calories, it isn't something you can burn with exercise. Eleven joggers with cholesterol levels of 185 - 330 died suddenly with severe coronary heart disease (J.A.M.A., 1982:247). A few years ago you may have heard of the tragic story of Jim Fixx, the author of several books on jogging. He died of a massive heart attack caused because his arteries were clogged with cholesterol. In his book he stated he ate at least three hamburgers and a milkshake before each marathon race because he believed he could burn it off with exercise. Unfortunately, Jim Fixx didn't realize cholesterol is not a substance that can be burned as calories, which is why his cholesterol level was 255 two weeks before he died. Jim refused to have a stress treadmill test because he believed he was in such great shape. You can feel good, look strong and fit, but you still will clog your arteries if you consume eggs, meat, cheese or butter daily.

WHAT IS CHOLESTEROL?

A study reported in The Archives of Internal Medicine, (Jan. 1990, Vol. 150) revealed 600 mg. of cholesterol (2 1/2 eggs) added to healthy men's diets, elevated the "bad" LDL cholesterol by as much as 25% (average 10%), independent of exercise and saturated fat. All of the men exercised regularly (aerobics 25 minutes per day, four times a week or more.) The exercise has no effect on preventing cholesterol added to the diet from building up in the bloodstream! This increase in cholesterol occurred even though they were consuming a diet low in saturated fat and less than 20% of total calories from fat. The study concluded that we must restrict our intake of dietary cholesterol to less than 200 mg. a day, even for people who exercise, follow a lowfat diet and avoid smoking. We at Delgado Medical advise zero and not more than 100 mg. of cholesterol per day in your diet.

The principal use of cholesterol is to make bile, an important digestive fluid that aids in the digestion of fat. Probably 70% of the total output of your cholesterol-making apparatus goes to bile. In the digestion process, bile is released into the small intestine to help you digest fat. As it goes through the small intestine the food gets digested, but the bile doesn't get reabsorbed until it reaches the ileum, at the very end of the small intestine (about 20 feet down the line). The ileum has something like a little vacuum cleaner which sucks up 90 to 95% of the bile and returns it to the liver. There it is regenerated and used to make more bile. So the body saves 90 to 95% of the bile that it makes. If it didn't, we'd have a tough time keeping up with the demand for bile and cholesterol.

The part of the bile that you lose (about 5 to 10%), passes into the large intestine and then out of the body through bowel movement. The bile that is excreted, since it is made principally from cholesterol, is the only way the body can lose cholesterol. If you didn't have this safety valve, in which you lose this little bit of bile every day, you couldn't eat any of the cholesterol foods. You would die at four years of age due to artery closure. In that situation, the body couldn't stand any cholesterol at all in the diet, and you'd be like the rabbit. The rabbit was apparently made to be solely a vegetable-eating animal. If it eats any animal protein at all, any cholesterol, its arteries will close fast - ten times faster than a man's arteries.

Man has a system that allows us to eat a small amount of cholesterol, but we cannot eat more than we lose in the bile that leaves our large intestine. That amount is equivalent to a daily ration of six oz. of meat, with small amounts of nonfat diary products. That is the maximum you can eat safely.

Even if you ate 25 eggs a day, your body would keep on making its own cholesterol as if you hadn't eaten any eggs at all! (Except a minor reduction in output by the body of 25%, or 250 mg., which is nearly equal to one egg yolk).

Eggs have one of the highest amounts of cholesterol of any food. One egg yolk has more cholesterol than a half pound of steak! Experiments have shown if chickens are fed eggs their arteries clog up with cholesterol within six months. This proves chickens can't even handle their own cholesterol. Eggs were intended to be an embryonic substance, and not for human consumption. Fertile eggs are just as dangerous as regular eggs and should not be eaten since the cholesterol is not "inactivated" as is believed by many people who have no scientific proof to make this claim. Eggs, cheese (cheese has twice the amount of cholesterol as red meat), butter and liver, are potent sources of cholesterol.

Find out your cholesterol level. If you haven't been tested yet, call our Delgado Medical Clinic in Fountain Valley at (714) 540-7725 for an appointment. If your cholesterol level is over 200, you're rapidly closing your arteries. If it's over 300, you have some very severely closed arteries, no matter how old you are. So we must bring these down to safe levels. Somewhere between 160 and 200 will stop further artery closure, while reversal of closure occurs best under 160. In countries where heart disease is unknown, cholesterol levels do not exceed 100 plus the individual's age, with a maximum of 160.

CHAPTER TWO
REDUCE YOUR CHOLESTEROL LEVEL SAVE YOUR LIFE

You will be surprised at how fast your cholesterol is going to drop by following the Delgado Program. Within two months, initial cholesterol levels of 160 drop 10%, the 220's drop 20%, and the 300's drop over 30%, all to safer levels.

Dr. Dean Ornish recently reported a study comparing patients placed on a zero cholesterol, low-fat (under 20% fat) Delgado-type of diet. The zero cholesterol low-fat diet substantially reduced plaque build up in each patient following this approach. However, patients following the outdated American Heart Association diet allowing 30% fat and 300 mg. of cholesterol increased plaque build up in the arteries according to before and after angiograms done on the patients by the end of the first year.

The serum cholesterol level will increase due to a high cholesterol diet. Other factors can elevate cholesterol levels, such as a low thyroid level, liver malfunction, weight gain, high triglyceride levels and several blood pressure and diabetic medications. The Delgado Plan with medical supervision, can help you to be free of most medications and control each of these factors. A zero cholesterol, low-fat diet will lower cholesterol for most people; but, a large drop in cholesterol level can be caused by factors other than dietary improvements. A decrease in serum cholesterol can be due to severe liver cell damage (caused by chemicals, drugs, hepatitis, the final stages of cancer, etc.), abnormally high thyroid levels, chronic anemia, cortisone and ACTH therapy or starvation. You should have blood tests to check for liver disorder, thyroid conditions or anemia if you're monitoring increased or decreased cholesterol levels that are caused by factors other than diet.

Provided the reduction in your blood cholesterol level is due to dietary changes, your blood cholesterol level will stay at the new lower level simply by consuming less than 100 mg. of cholesterol a day, and by eating water-soluble fibers found in oat bran, corn flakes, black-eyed peas, carrots, etc. After about four months, the blood cholesterol starts to go up temporarily while the plaques are dissolving. Don't get discouraged, stay with the program and within several months you'll have an ideal cholesterol level. (Some people with very high initial levels may take nearly three to six years to reduce their cholesterol below 200, and finally to under 160).

A book titled Heart Failure by Thomas Moore, former campaign manager for Gary Hart and newpaper writer, has misled people into believing a low cholesterol level (under 160), will lead to an increased risk of stroke, gallstones and colon cancer. His misrepresentation of the facts begins with studies based on the Northern Japanese high rate of stroke that he relates to their low cholesterol level. There are two different types of strokes. One is related to atherosclerosis or blocked arteries causing brain damage. The second type of stroke (hemorrhagic) results from hypertensive pressure, causing arterial blow-out. The truth is the Northern Japanese people use more salt than any culture in the world, resulting in high blood pressure, a well known cause of hemorrhagic stroke. The Southern Japanese have a low cholesterol level, a lower sodium intake and a low incidence of atherosclerotic and hemorrhagic stroke. Worldwide people with the lowest cholesterol have among the lowest rate of stroke related to atherosclerotic plaques.

Thomas Moore also asserts that according to the Veterans Administration Study, men with low cholesterol levels had the highest rate of gallstones and colon cancer. What he neglected to explain was that the high consumption of polyunsaturated oils used in the studies to lower cholesterol tend to form gallstones and increase the risk of colon cancer. This study also included up to 300 mg. of dietary cholesterol per day. This dangerous combination of polyunsaturated fats and cholesterol is a well known promoter of gallstones and cancer. People who follow a diet of less than 20% fat and under 100 mg. of cholesterol per day, have a low incidence of gallstones and colon cancer.

Delgado Medical has checked over 20,000 people from June 1985 to June 1987 (new patients and seminar attendees) for cholesterol levels. Of that number, 95% had a cholesterol level exceeding 160 mg. (the safe range is 100 to 160) and more than 50% had dangerous cholesterol levels of over 200 mg/dl!

Many patients, though, are erroneously told that their cholesterol level is in the normal range. But it's not a "normal range." Those numbers are simply the average range for this already very sick American population with atherosclerosis. Labs determined so-called normal cholesterol levels by taking a group of 1,000 people of each decade of age (10-20, 20-30, 30-40, etc.) who exhibited no symptoms of illness or disease, and testing their cholesterol levels. What the researchers failed to consider was that people showing no symptoms can already have significant plaque build-up and artery closure. As a result, your arteries can be 90% closed and yet you're considered normal. So, when we take 1,000 people like this, their cholesterol levels come out to be 160 to 320, and that is a so-called "normal" range for the American population!

REDUCE YOUR CHOLESTEROL

When the Cleveland Clinic examined the cholesterol levels of over 1,000 people in the so-called normal range, and compared the results to their angiograms, almost every person had serious artery closure of coronary arteries. The large Framingham Massachusetts Study has been monitoring 5200 people since 1948. They found that if the cholesterol level is over 260, there is a 400% greater incidence of heart disease-caused death than if the cholesterol is less than 220. As a result, we must lower our cholesterol levels to optimum ranges.

The Centers for Disease Control released this statement in February of 1984 to laboratories across the country:

DEAR DOCTOR,

THE STANDARD LABORATORY PRACTICE OF INDICATING A NORMAL RANGE OF LAB VALUES MAY HAVE BECOME MISLEADING IN THE CASE OF SERUM CHOLESTEROL LEVELS. THERE IS NOW CONVINCING EVIDENCE THAT THIS SO-CALLED "NORMAL" RANGE FOR CHOLESTEROL, BASED ON AVERAGE LEVELS IN THE U.S., MAY BE CONSIDERABLY HIGHER THAN THE OPTIMAL RANGE, ABOVE WHICH THE RISK OF CORONARY HEART DISEASE INCREASES.

THE ADVISORY PANEL OF THE COUNCIL ON SCIENTIFIC AFFAIRS RECOMMENDS THAT "CHOLESTEROL LEVELS ABOVE 194 MG . . . DESERVE TREATMENT. THE CRITICAL LEVELS FOR WOMEN ARE EVEN LOWER (J.A.M.A. 250:1873 '83). RECENT STUDIES SHOW THAT REDUCING HYPER-CHOLESTEROLEMIA REDUCES THE INCIDENCE OF CORONARY HEART DISEASE . . ."

Women are also at great danger. The International Atherosclerosis Project compared autopsy reports on 3,000 deceased women from different areas of the world. They found that premenopausal women in some areas had more atherosclerosis than men who lived in other parts of the world.

White American women aged 35 to 45 are twice as likely to die of heart disease as are Japanese men of the same age. Yet, American women smoke far less than the Japanese men. The higher cholesterol levels of American women stand accused. White women in the U.S. had 3 times as much severe plaque as women of the same age living in countries who eat much less cholesterol in their diets. American black women had as much advanced atherosclerosis as American black men. The only reason that white women have less atherosclerosis before menopause than white men is not because of a hormone difference, but rather a dietary difference of slightly less eggs, cheese and meat intake than men.

Dr. Kaare Norum of the University of Oslo School of Medicine polled 200 top world scientists who had attended heart disease conferences. He found a full 92% recommended reducing cholesterol and fat in the diet, while simultaneously changing their eating habits.

The dairy farmers, wanting in recent years to silence the American Heart Association, filed a multimillion dollar lawsuit. The farmers stated that they would not support the efforts of the local Wisconsin Heart Association Chapter to raise money in a dairy state. Apparently their threats proved effective, because the result was that diet information is now available only on request, and the Dairy Council diet advice is also included with the Heart Association reply.

In 1974 the National Academy of Sciences advised that eggs no longer be used as the protein standard, since new research suggests egg protein is not as ideal as once thought. However, this information has been suppressed and ignored. The proteins found in whole grains, rice, wheat and oats provide the best sources for humans. Eggs, meat and cheese are better for carnivores like rats, dogs and cats.

The National Heart, Lung and Blood Institute (NHLBI) criticized two studies funded by the egg industry that appeared to show that eggs have no effect on blood cholesterol. Dr. Margaret Flynn, University of Missouri, and Drs. Grant Slater and Alfin Slater of UCLA reported that adding cholesterol to a normal diet (already high in cholesterol) wasn't significant. However, "despite the author's conclusions and all the serious flaws in the study, the results do show an effect of egg cholesterol on plasma (blood) cholesterol," said the NHLBI.

The UCLA study has received widespread publicity - and apparently not by accident. The California Egg Program (egg growers) paid for the study and assigned its advertising agency to publicize the results. The agency did its job well, generating publicity through news conferences, radio and TV interviews, and an ingenious plan of inserting 3 millions flyers into egg cartons.

According to Dr. Jean Mayer, a respected nutritionist, "the consumption of large amounts of dietary cholesterol still increases blood cholesterol," though the body can reduce its own production of cholesterol by 25% of its 1000 mg. output per day. But when the average American eats over 600 mg. of cholesterol per day, obviously the 250 mg. drop in production is still not enough (350 mg. short, to be exact) to compensate fully. Cholesterol from the diet more than 100 mg. a day has become our country's principal cause of premature death, with over one million people dying every year.

The largest and best control study on dietary cholesterol and heart attack risk was conducted on 3,806 people over an eight year period. The Journal of American Medical Association (1984: 251:351-364) proved conclusively that a reduction of dietary cholesterol can reduce blood cholesterol and dramatically cut the death rate from premature death due to heart attacks and atherosclerosis.

Dr. Charles Glueck is the Director of the University of Cincinnati Lipid Research Center, one of twelve centers that participated in the project. He reported, "For every 1% reduction in total cholesterol level, there is a 2% reduction of heart disease risk." This, says Project Director Basil Rifkind, is the evidence scientists have been waiting for. "It is a turning point in cholesterol - heart disease research."

Dr. Antonio Gotto, President of the American Heart Association, explains that since atherosclerosis develops slowly throughout life, children should be started on a low-fat and low-cholesterol diet at the age of two (right after weaning). The U.S. Department of Health, after examining 6,000 children (ages 1-17), concluded that over 60% of the U.S. children have cholesterol levels over 160 by age 3, and 10% already have a cholesterol level over 200.

Dr. William Castelli is the Director of the Framingham Study for the National Institute of Health and lecturer at Harvard Medical School. He not only wants to reduce the risk of heart disease, but once a person is diagnosed with advanced hardening of the arteries, Dr. Castelli believes that using a Delgado-type diet the patient can strive to reverse and dissolve the disease. He says, "The timetable for reversibility goes like this: The fatty cellular deposits will actually go away in a matter of weeks; the extra-cellular fat takes up to a year and a half; the fibrous lesion is the hardest thing to remove, and that takes up to four years. To see massive reversibility, we need to get cholesterol levels down below 150. If we do that, we are going to see a lot of reversibility. A level of 170 or 180 isn't as safe as many people in this country think; but if we did get people down to 170, they would certainly do better." Probably half them would reverse. If you want to talk about 90% reversibility, you've got to get people's cholesterol count below 150."

Why have our drug experiments failed? They reduce risk, but haven't reduced plaques as effectively. These drugs only reduce cholesterol by 10%. No miracles happen at 10%. Some people improve, but if we want to start seeing this situation turn around, we all have a lot more work to do than we've done so far in this country. And the first step is diet.

In the average American hospital, the diet kitchen is run by the same companies who service all the local hotels. For the people who have bypass surgery, what do you think they have for breakfast on the morning after surgery? Bacon and eggs! Robert Wissler, M.D., famous pathologist at the University of Chicago, took the patients' house diet at Billings Hospital and fed it to his baboons: they all lost their legs from atherosclerosis. We need a diet-learning center in every hospital in every town in America. We need to start teaching low-fat nutrition in schools and colleges - straight through all stages of life, and we haven't done that. We have very powerful lobbies in this country preventing the masses of people from learning the truth about proper nutrition.

In Europe, on a wartime diet of rationing, atherosclerosis was gone in two years. In fact, during this time the European universities couldn't find even one case of atherosclerosis to show the medical students how horrible lesions look. Yet two years before any autopsy case would have shown these lesions.

The medical journal Circulation (Vol. 64, July 1981, No. 1) reported 32 angiographically-documented cases of regression of human atherosclerosis. They state atherosclerosis is almost completely preventable and it is substantially reversible.

The body loses a small amount (100 mg.) of cholesterol daily with the bowel movements as bile. In one to three years you could get rid of 36,000 to 100,000 mg., which is enough to clean up your arteries at the rate of 10% a year and be free of 30% or more of the plaques. To reverse (dissolve) atherosclerotic plaques, follow the Delgado Program of nutrition, exercise and stress management, which is medically monitored by our clinic in Fountain Valley.

REDUCE BAD LDL CHOLESTEROL, DON'T WORRY ABOUT GOOD HDL

Cholesterol is made up of different components called lipoproteins such as HDL, LDL and VLDL. Don't be confused or misled by doctors saying that the ratio of HDL to total cholesterol is more important than the total cholesterol level. The only cases where cholesterol of 180 or 190 are acceptable would be in certain women who have a high HDL level of about 80. If the LDL is less than 95 it's considered safer than if the LDL is above 95.

Our program will reduce the "bad" LDL (low density lipoprotein) cholesterol, which causes hardening of the arteries, while raising the "good" HDL (high density lipoprotein) cholesterol, which removes the plaque build-up in the arteries. The VLDL transports triglycerides from the liver to tissues where they form pockets of fat. Once the VLDL's have dumped their load of triglycerides, they become LDL's and begin carrying cholesterol from the liver to cells around the body (VLDL levels should be under 40). If your VLDL is above 40, The Delgado Program will help to lower VLDL's as you lower triglycerides.

People are born with nearly equal amounts of HDL and LDL, producing a natural 1 to 1 ratio

(VLDL makes up the remainder). Yet, if your cholesterol level is higher than 160 mg., the HDL will not protect you any longer, as shown by comparing people in Japan to those in Finland who had equally high "good" HDL's. The Japanese were free of heart disease and had 140 total cholesterol levels, as opposed to the Finnish who had high total cholesterol levels leading to a high death rate from heart disease. The extensive Framingham Study also confirmed that higher HDL levels are not protective against high LDL's (Lancet, Sept. 20,'80, p.604, Ancel Keys). Most people in the U.S. have a ratio of 1 HDL to 4 LDL, caused by eating more cholesterol than the body can excrete.

The Delgado Program will help you to reduce this ratio to a more favorable equal ratio, similar to what it was when you were a newborn infant. During the first six weeks your total cholesterol level will drop because the "bad" LDL is rapidly being removed from the body. The "good" HDL will come down slightly, and then gradually rise with daily exercise. HDL cholesterol levels will automatically be lower in people following a low-fat, high carbohydrate diet. You and your doctor should not be concerned about having a low HDL level when following this diet. According to Practical Cardiology, Vol. 15, No. 40, Oct. 1989, "fresh HDL is still being produced normally and is doing its job well . . . because old HDL is being cleared away more efficiently by this type of diet." Your HDL level may range between 25 - 40, a level previously thought to be too low, but here it is desirable.

The Tarahumara Indians, who are free of heart disease, were found to have low HDL levels (25 - 35 mg./dl) and a total cholesterol of 125 mg. for all ages (children to senior citizens). They eat beans, tortillas, vegetables, cereals and fruits (American Journal Clinical Nutrition, 35: April '82).

The Eskimos have been mistakenly identified as a high fat-eating culture, yet in Scientific American, Sept. 1971, it was found that Central Arctic Eskimos actually eat a lower cholesterol, lower-in-fat diet (under 23% fat) compared to our intake. This is why the Eskimos living in the central arctic region have no heart disease. However, Eskimos living in the coastal regions who eat blubber (animal fat) in large amounts do have a high rate of heart disease.

The Masai tribe in Africa was examined in 1962 by Dr. Mann, whose research was sponsored by the American Meat Association. It was believed that they were free of coronary artery disease (according to stress treadmill tests), though they ate high cholesterol foods - almost entirely meat, blood of cows and sour milk. So, for ten years the Meat

Association said there was no need to change the American diet. In response, Dr. Mann cautioned that we shouldn't make such claims, until we do autopsies on Masai who died accidentally.

Finally, in 1972, the American Meat Association agreed to sponsor a new study to include 50 autopsies. I think that is the last study they will ever sponsor because they found that the Masai had the most massive plaques they had ever seen in people of similar ages. But you ask, how could they pass the treadmill test? Because the Masai walk at a fast pace over thirty miles a day herding cattle and visiting friends. Their coronary arteries were found to have enlarged to twice the size of those of a normal person. Also, it was discovered that the large amount of sour milk they drank apparently artificially kept their blood cholesterol at a low level of 120 mg., while pushing cholesterol into their arteries. So, though they passed the treadmill test (because of their enlarged blood flow), they still were in danger of plaques breaking off and traveling upstream to cause stroke or death. Cultures in the world that are protected from cholesterol build-up in the arteries follow a Delgado-type of health plan: low in fat, low in cholesterol and rich in complex carbohydrates.

CHAPTER THREE
WINNING THE BATTLE AGAINST CHOLESTEROL

Cholesterol is the leading cause of heart disease, ahead of cigarette smoking, high blood pressure, stress and obesity, according to Dr. Stephen Hulley, professor of medicine at U.C. San Francisco. Quitting smoking was the second most important factor that helped reduce hardening of the arteries. One hundred forty-four thousand people's lives were saved by smoking cessation (1984 statistics). These people were saved because they were no longer exposed to so much carbon monoxide in smoke that accelerated the buildup of cholesterol in the arteries.

The National Institute for Health (NIH) reported Dec. 13, 1984, that it has been "established beyond a reasonable doubt" that reducing elevated levels of cholesterol in the bloodstream will lower the risk of heart attacks.

The NIH team of experts said all Americans past the age of two should adopt a diet with sharply reduced cholesterol and fat intakes. (This conclusion was based on a review of research studies primarily sponsored by taxpayer money). Food companies should be encouraged to intensify efforts to develop and sell foods with reduced cholesterol and fat content. At this time food labels show the amount of fat per grams. However, they rarely list the cholesterol content.

The NIH panel said, "It is staggering to realize" that about half the U.S. population has cholesterol levels for which "most would agree there is an increased risk of developing premature coronary heart disease." Dr. Steinberg, panel chairman, also added, "And the cholesterol levels of many more Americans, while not in the high risk category, may still pose some heart disease dangers."

Over 60% of the U.S. population has a cholesterol level higher than 200 mg., while only 5% has the ideal level of under 150 mg. Public education, such as the Delgado Medical Program, is vital so that high-risk people can be quickly identified and treated. Dr. Steinberg, professor of medicine at U.C. San Diego, states "We hope that five years from now people will say, 'I better go get my cholesterol checked.'"

I have conducted many seminars and at every one, I ask the question, "How many people here do not know their cholesterol level?" I have found 70 to 90% of the people in the audiences do not even know their cholesterol level. But, I am proud to say that of those people who join The Delgado Program, a majority not only know their cholesterol level, but have lowered their cholesterol levels an average of

20% within eight weeks after starting the program.

We must turn to nutrition and prevention if we are going to be successful in curing heart disease. The number of coronary bypass operations being done now exceeds 160,000 a year. This makes it the nations's leading surgical procedure. At a cost of $25,000 per operation, this makes a grand total of over two billion dollars per year spent on bypass surgery alone. Yet when the NIH released the results of the longest study on bypass surgery ever conducted (ten thousand patients treated surgically were compared to ten thousand patients treated with medication only), it was found there was a decrease in survival rate in the surgery group by 1%. In addition, there was no difference in the amount or type of recreational activity either group later engaged in, or in the number of each group who returned to work.

We must accept the notion that coronary artery closure is mostly a nutritional disease and that it will respond to food and fitness measures. In London, England, since 1981 seven hospitals have switched to the high-complex carbohydrate, low-fat diet recommended by the British Medical Aspects of Food Policy, and have found health food is practical, popular (sales in the staff cafeteria have gone up 60% since being introduced) and saves money. The hospital group economizes on the food bill and saves over $8,000 per year by eliminating the need for laxatives. Typical foods now served in the London hospital group include brown rice with peas, baked sweet potatoes, watermelon, wholemeal bread, low-fat cheese, lentils, kidney beans, black-eyed peas, barley in soup, skim milk and grilled fish (not fried). In addition, they have greatly reduced the usage of oils, salt and sugar.

According to a nationwide Department of Health survey done in 1980, over one-third (36%) of the cholesterol consumed in our country came from eggs, followed by beefsteak and hamburgers (16%), whole milk and cheese (6%), and hot dogs, ham and bologna (4%). Fortunately over 90% of the 10,000 people who attended our orientation meetings in 1990 dramatically reduced meat and cheese intake and stopped eating eggs every week! You should never eat egg yolks, now that you know each yolk has 212 mg. of cholesterol and that your body can only excrete 100 mg. a day (according to the 1985 Nobel Prize for Medicine recipients, Drs. Brown and Goldstein).

We've heard people say, "I tried to lower my cholesterol level by giving up red meat for chicken and fish, and I eat only 1 egg per week. My level didn't go down at all. Some doctors and dieticians say I have a genetic problem and I'm incurable."

Our response is only 1 in 1,000,000 (a total of only 230 Americans) have a possible genetic malfunction of the liver, and if this was your problem, by the age of 10 you would've had a heart attack, or at least a cholesterol level of over 500. The Annals of Internal Medicine, 1988; Vol. 108, reported the case of a 12 year old boy who had a genetic malfunction of the liver, resulting in a cholesterol level of 1160, an LDL of 1103, and severly clogged arteries. A heart transplant was done that temporarily provided new circulation to his heart. Next, a liver transplant successfully reduced his cholesterol level down to 200 in two months on an unrestricted diet. After all the effort, it's unfortunate the doctor didn't even recommend a change in diet! He was saved at the age of 12 and likely to die by the age of 45, not from tissue rejection, but from dietary causes. The solution to most people's cholesterol problem is to avoid egg yolks altogether, and to realize even the white part of chicken, fish or turkey has nearly the same amount of cholesterol as does red meat. You need to cut back on your total meat intake (chicken, fish, turkey, red meat, etc.) to no more than three 6-ounce servings per week.

WHERE CHOLESTEROL IS FOUND AND HOW TO GET RID OF IT

CHOLESTEROL CONTENT 3 1/2 OUNCES

ANIMAL PROTEIN VS. PLANT FOOD

Animal protein		Plant food	
Egg yolks	1,500 mg.	Oatmeal	0 mg.
Whole eggs	500 mg.	Rice	0 mg.
Liver (beef)	300 mg.	Wheat	0 mg.
Butter	250 mg.	Cantaloupe	0 mg.
Shrimp	160 mg.	Bananas	0 mg.
Cheese, crab	100 mg.	Orange	0 mg.
Fish (mackerel)	95 mg.	Corn	0 mg.
Veal	90 mg.	Potato	0 mg.
Turkey, lobster	82 mg.	Squash	0 mg.
Beef, pork, lamb, salmon	68 mg.	Split peas	0 mg.
Tuna (in water)	63 mg.	Pinto beans	0 mg.
Chicken	60 mg.	Garbanzos	0 mg.
Scallops,	52 mg.	Blackeyed peas	0 mg.
Clams	49 mg.	Nuts	0 mg.
Milk, whole	11 mg.	Seeds	0 mg.
Milk, skimmed	3 mg.	Rice milk	0 mg.

ALL ANIMAL PRODUCTS CONTAIN CHOLESTEROL.

ALL GRAINS, FRUITS, VEGETABLES, LEGUMES, NUTS AND SEEDS CONTAIN NO CHOLESTEROL.

THE BATTLE AGAINST CHOLESTEROL

SUMMARY TO PREVENT OR REDUCE ATHEROSCLEROSIS

The following information could save your life, and the lives of your loved ones, without the potentially harmful side effects of drugs or mega dosages of supplements.

Study the list of foods that contain cholesterol, and work toward reducing your intake of cholesterol to less than 100 mg. a day.

Be sure to avoid obvious sources of unneeded dietary cholesterol by using egg whites or Egg Beaters instead of egg yolks; use Lifetime cheese that is 50% lower in cholesterol and fat than regular cheese; use grains, beans, vegetable and fruit in place of organ meats, shell fish, poultry, fish, beef or pork; use Butter Buds, Molly McButter or apple butter instead of butter, rice milk in place of whole or skim milk; use smaller amounts of lean meats like halibut, scallops, clams, sole, turkey or chicken (under two oz. per day.) Try not eating meat at least three or more days a week.

TO RAPIDLY REDUCE YOUR CHOLESTEROL LEVEL, PREPARE YOUR MEALS WITHOUT ANY TYPE OF MEAT AS OFTEN AS POSSIBLE.

If the food originated from an animal of any type, it contains cholesterol. Even the white part of the chicken without the skin has cholesterol permeated throughout it. Tuna or turkey has as much cholesterol as red meat, so eat it in moderation. Have you tried our recipes for wheat meat, bean or vegetable sandwiches instead of tuna or turkey sandwiches? I'm sure you'll grow to enjoy them as I have.

Eat more water soluble fiber (pectin, guar and bengal gum) foods, which soak up bile and cholesterol in your intestines like a sponge. This helps to remove cholesterol from your body in the bowel movements.

The foods that lower cholesterol best include black-eyed peas, kidney, pinto and navy beans, broccoli, green peas, carrots, chinese cabbage, sweet potatoes, corn, corn meal, rolled oats, apples and prunes.

Pectin fiber in grapefruit, apples, applesauce and prunes eaten daily will accelerate the removal of cholesterol. The special fiber in broccoli, zucchini, squash, cauliflower, carrots, potatoes, artichokes and Chinese cabbage can lower cholesterol and help you to lose weight when added daily to a large vegetable salad, casseroles or soups.

THE BATTLE AGAINST CHOLESTEROL

Eat 1 cup a day of black-eyed peas - cooked fresh, frozen or canned. Black-eyed peas have a large amount of soluble fiber to reduce cholesterol. You can add the black-eyed peas to a vegetable soup if you need to lose weight, since soups are filling and satisfying, and great for weight loss. You may use other beans (such as pinto, navy, etc.) or green peas as well for added benefit.

According to the American Journal of Clinical Nutrition (Vol. 34:824, 1981) over 15 grams of soluble fiber from certain foods can accelerate the removal of cholesterol from your intestines. For example, to help your body to remove excess cholesterol, you could eat one cup of black-eyed peas, one bowl of oatmeal, one cup of corn and one pear that would equal 11.5 + 3.5 + 1 = 17.8 grams. The foods listed my book "Weight Loss and Energy Now" in the Composition of Foods section have been analyzed using new methods to show the amount of water soluble fiber they contain.

Analyze your diet. Are you getting seven to fifteen grams of soluble fiber each day to help lower your cholesterol level?

A study in the New England Journal of Medicine 1990; 322, revealed that oat bran, as compared to Cream of Wheat, only lowers cholesterol by 3% in patients with initially low cholesterol levels. This reduction in cholesterol is not much; but, when added to the total Delgado plan you will see good results. If you decide to use oatbran, be sure to avoid products that have added oils, egg yolks or sugar.

Psyllium Husk or Seed (Metamucil) is one of the highest sources of soluble fiber. Psyllium husk is a soluble fiber from the coating of seeds of blond psyllium in the sunflower family, and can dramatically reduce your cholesterol level. According to Dr. James Anderson, psyllium husk is cheaper and safer than drugs like cholestyramine, and lowers cholesterol just as well. Add two to six tablespoons of psyllium husk or Metamucil to your cereal or juice. The psyllium flakes turn into a gel when mixed with cereal and water or fruit juice. Psyllium husk is available at Delgado Medical, health food stores or as Metamucil at pharmacies.

In summary to reduce your cholesterol effectively:

1. Eat mainly foods that have roots and grew like grains, beans, fruits, vegetables and sprouts containing absolutely no cholesterol.

2. Minimize the intake of foods that have legs, wings or tails and could wiggle or move like meat or dairy products to less than six ounces (100 mg. of cholesterol) no more than three times per week.

3. Eat at least 15 grams of soluble fiber each day from oats, corn, beans, or certain fruits.

If your cholesterol does not come down:

4. Add three to six tablespoons of psyllium husk divided in half, morning and night to your cereals, juice or water.

5. Make an appointment to see one of our doctors in Fountain Valley at Delgado Medical or see your doctor to rule out any liver or thyroid disorders, hormone imbalances, side effects from medications you may be taking or diseases that are known to affect cholesterol levels.

We are often asked about supplements to lower cholesterol. As of this writing both Drs. Leaf and Connors, who have studied the effect of fish oil products, are opposed to their use. Dr. Connors states, "We do not recommend that people take codliver oil . . . avoid EPA-Omega-3 fatty acid fish oil or DHA, since their safety has not been established." Avoid fish oil (Omega-3) since it contains cholesterol. It may elevate your cholesterol level the way it has in over one-third of the people taking it in recent studies. Fish oil is 100% fat and taking too much could elevate your triglyceride level.

We also are concerned because pollutants like PCB's or Mercury can concentrate in the flesh of fish, and may show up in the fish oil. Finally, excessive thinning of blood platelets caused by fish oil may be associated with the reports of Eskimos having an increased death rate from stroke.

There are ways to lower cholesterol levels that do not increase the excretion of cholesterol out of the body, but these methods may worsen the problem. Some people are taking lecithin (which is 100% fat) to try to reduce their cholesterol levels. However, when lecithin was given to young men it actually raised fat levels in the blood, lowered lung function and created red blood clusters that lasted several days!

Dr. Meyer Friedman warned that lecithin could raise serum cholesterol even higher and deposit even more atherosclerosis, according to his book, Pathogenesis of Coronary Artery Disease. You should avoid lecithin. Lecithin is of no value to the body, according to Dr. Connors, because it is completely digested in the intestines. Therefore, it cannot emulsify or dissolve fat and cholesterol in the blood.

Vegetable oils such as corn oil have been found to reduce blood cholesterol also, but since there is no increase in excretion out of the body, it has been concluded that the cholesterol has been pushed into the arteries, according to Dr. Ahrens.

Many people are using niacin to lower cholesterol. Caution is advised against the use of mega dosages (three to six grams) of the vitamin niacin or nicotinic acid. It could dilate the blood vessels in the eyes leading to blurred vision and possible hemorrhages in the eyes in susceptible people. Other possible side effects that have been reported in the Journal of the American Medical Association from the Coronary Drug Project include: irregular heartbeat, increases in uric acid and gout, elevation in glucose and worsening of diabetes, flushed skin leading to possible frostbite in cold weather, gastric upset and peptic ulcers, an itching rash (which goes away only when you stop taking high dosages of niacin) and worsening of liver disease.

There are several drugs that lower cholesterol. However, all have been shown to have various negative side effects. You can check with one of our doctors for guidance in this regard.

BLOOD TEST RESULTS ON DELGADO HEALTH PLAN

Your drop in cholesterol may be as much as 20% in only three weeks. And, with continued treatment following the Delgado Plan for over one year, your level may continue to nudge down. Remember, your tissues and arteries are probably saturated with cholesterol.

During this time your blood cholesterol level probably will stabilize (although it can go up while it's drawing cholesterol out of your arteries and tissues.) Therefore, it may take from one to five years before you drain out most of the cholesterol build-up. This could help you avoid future vascular accidents, surgery or loss of function (hearing, sight, sexual function.) You should have your cholesterol level checked every three to six weeks until it reaches an ideal level of less than 160.

If your cholesterol level starts out at 240 or higher, it can drop to as low as 190 in only three weeks. Then it may stay between 190 and 220 for several years before it finally drops below 160. Don't be discouraged, because this draining out period is common and to be expected. Consider how many years of your life you ate foods concentrated in cholesterol. It is going to take time to drain the excess from the walls of your arteries and tissues. But, you have stopped adding to the build-up of cholesterol and quality years of life are being gained as you improve every day. Eventually you will be excited to find that your cholesterol level will reduce below 160 as you follow the Delgado Plan.

You also can watch for a rapid drop in the "bad" LDL cholesterol in your blood, and a stabilization of the "good" HDL cholesterol.

NICK DELGADO'S RESULTS

The following chart represents a detailed account of Nick Delgado's blood lipids during the last ten years:

	Cholesterol	LDL	HDL	VLDL
8-18-80 Jennings Lab	126	-	-	-
6-11-82 Bioscience Lab	146	101	33	12
9-26-85 Naples Lab	154	83	48	23
10-11-86 Naples Lab	142	87	40	14
6-5-87 Naples Lab	131	104	22	4
10-26-87 C.R.L.	107	60	29	17
11-4-90 National Lab	145	90	36	29
4-17-92 S.D.L.				

Cholesterol continues to be betwen 100-150 and triglycerides are routinely under 100.

NOTE: My blood testing was done in a non-fasting state. Eating low-fat, high carbohydrate foods and following a daily, mild exercise program on the Delgado Plan has allowed me to maintain remarkably healthy blood test results over the years. Nonfasting (taking blood after eating) gives results based on your true state of health. Fasting gives artificially low levels especially after eating for triglyceride and glucose. These low levels obtained after fasting twelve hours will give a patient a false sense of security. I challenge you to have your blood tests during the normal course of the day after eating. If you have abnormally high results, you probably have developed eating habits and patterns that require major improvements as offered by The Delgado Plan.

CHOLESTEROL

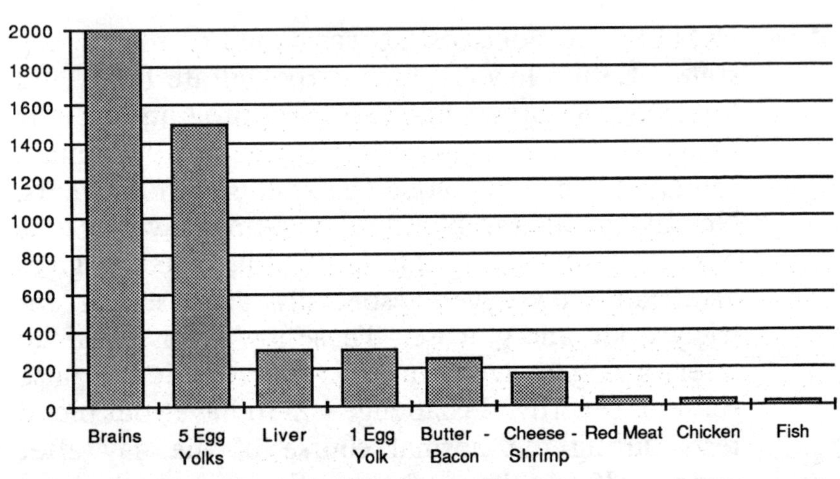

Cholesterol in 3 1/2 oz. (100 grams) of food (Shown in Mg.)

0 mg.:

Grains, Beans, Nuts, Seeds, Fruits and Vegetables

CHAPTER FOUR

ESTABLISHING GOALS

To accomplish your goals, you need to establish them at the beginning of your self-improvement program. In other words, write down your goals. What are they, especially in the area of health? Also, what are your goals in business, relationships, etc.? I keep a calendar on which I enter all the different goals I want to accomplish each day. As these goals are reached, I cross them off my list. By the end of the day, if there are certain goals I did not complete, I simply assign them to the very next day. My calendar is filled with short and long term goals that are prioritized according to life values. In the past, when I read a book, I would write down goals on the inside jacket that I wanted to do during my life. I enjoy looking back into these old books because I find the goals I had written have been accomplished and sometimes even surpassed. I now keep a daily journal of future goals, plans and appointments. Writing down your goals is extremely important.

The next important stage is to gain the knowledge to attain your goals. This is what is being done in the area of health through our tapes and books. We are giving you the knowledge. Now you must use this knowledge and take action.

Probably the most important step in the area of goals is taking action. Taking action means simply "DO IT!" Apply what you have learned. This will work for you. For example, we are giving you certain recommendations for items to obtain. Now it is up to you to find that jogger and have it for your use. Make that trip to the supermarket or health food store and stock your pantry and refrigerator with the foods that cause you to lose weight and to improve your health.

The final step is to reward yourself after you have accomplished these efforts. Rewards are very important. Think of some examples. The first reward that usually comes to mind is FOOD. Food could be considered a reward, but if you use the wrong foods you will be defeating your efforts. I was asked what are the foods I miss most often. I used to eat steak, but now when I think about it, it does not appeal to me. It doesn't have the satisfying taste that it used to have. I just do not enjoy it anymore. I used to eat large amounts of cheese, but when I tasted it again after such a long time, it tasted very fatty to me. I now associate extreme fatigue with the taste of cheese, meat or oils and this helps me to avoid them. What I have enjoyed in my new eating lifestyle is a variety of ethnic foods. I have frequented a variety of Thai, Chinese, Vietnamese, Japanese, Italian and Mexican restaurants. One of the rewards I enjoy is tasting new cuisines by taking my family out to eat.

Frequently the reward suggested by my class members is clothing. In the area of success when you dress appropriately you have a better chance of attaining your success goals. Entertainment is another type of reward: movies, plays, games or even vacations are all good therapy. There are many places that may be enjoyed - the beach, the mountains, the desert, etc. As suggested by my class members, sex also can be an excellent reward. You can begin to form a positive association of motivation by including rewards you enjoy to reinforce your accomplished goals.

Some people, though, seem concerned that when they are working hard toward achieving their goals, they are doing too much. So they ask, "Is this really worthwhile?" After you have worked hard enough you can allow yourself to sit back and enjoy the rewards of your hard efforts. Let's face it, we all have to put in that hard work before we can become successful. You must give that extra effort in the early stages of your pursuit of your goals to keep things flowing, otherwise all your efforts will have been lost.

Surround yourself with positive people and input. When you are around negative individuals, their negative ideas are easily digested. You may even begin to think negatively yourself. It is much easier to achieve a positive success attitude if you are around positive people who encourage you to lose weight and improve your health. You can really begin to do it. Start this week by making friends with or reuniting with successful, positive people and applying positive methods.

Positive methods may include reading success books or listening to motivational cassette tapes. There comes a day when your car breaks down, you're late for an appointment and you lose a contract. By the end of the day you are not feeling well. Everything seems to be falling apart. You feel you are never going to make it. At that point, take a moment, but just a moment, to be immobilized. Now pick yourself up and think positive and start out again.

At the point of being immobilized, you may need something external to help you. Take out that positive book or cassette. One of the most positive individuals that can be suggested is Zig Ziglar. His book, SEE YOU AT THE TOP, will enrich your life beyond imagination. He mentions some very important factors to achieving success. Zig Ziglar has motivated me in my personal life as much as any other success motivator. I suggest you have your bookstore order this book for you if they are out of stock. He also has cassette tapes available. Other motivating individuals are Robert Schuller, Greg Laurie, Norman Vincent Peale, Michael Korda, Wayne Dyer, Brian Tracy and Tony Robbins.

I personally have a library containing over one thousand cassette tapes and I subscribe to weekly tape services. I enjoy listening to these while I'm on the road. Often after long drives, I will continue to sit in my car after I have arrived at my destination, waiting to hear the end of a tape because of the enjoyment I get in listening to these motivating individuals. I believe this type of tape may be of help to you also. Everyone who attends our seminars and achieves the benefits, maintains a high level of motivation and a positive attitude over the long term by following these steps:

1. Use our cassette tapes, videos and books to feed your mind and improve your expertise.
2. Keep a goal planner journal.
3. Associate with positive, successful people for role models.

DIET AND EXERCISE PLANNING CALENDAR

Sunday	Monday	Tuesday	Wednesday	Thursday	Friday	Saturday

Make Your Own Calendar For Future Months

- *Write in the type and length of exercise (your goal is 30 minutes, 6 times a week). Note your pulse rate count.*
- *List what you're eating.*
- *Hours of sleep, how you feel.*

Example

Walked with heavy hands.
30 min., pulse 120.
Grain cereal.
Banana.
Salad bar, Fruit
Veggie soup
Rice casserole
Potatoes, bread
7 hours sleep
Feel great!

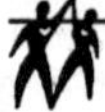

CHAPTER FIVE

IMPORTANCE OF A HEALTHY LIFESTYLE

One of the most important desires we all have is to live a longer, healthier life. If we look throughout the world, we find groups of people who achieve this Optimum Health.

After visiting the Hunzas of Pakistan, Dr. Alexander Leaf, Chief of Medical Services at Massachusetts Medical School, said, "It is the fitness of the elderly rather than their age that impresses me." The Hunzukuts play a violent, fast-moving form of polo and volleyball in which 70-year-old men are playing alongside young boys.

Dr. Samuel Rosen of Mt. Sinai Hospital in New York found upon medical examination that the Hunzas have remarkably acute hearing past the age of 65. These people also have their teeth, luxuriant hair, good eyesight, and erect posture. They are free of degenerative diseases like hardening of the arteries or heart disease, diabetes, hypertension, cancer and arthritis.

There are also other groups of people possessing remarkable health. One such group, the Tarahumaras (foot runners) of Chuhuahua, Mexico, play an extraordinary game of kickball that takes 48 hours of nonstop running over a distance of 180 miles!

In Ecuador, Dr. Miguel Salvador, leader of a medical team examining the Vilcabamban Indians, found a total absence of serious ailments, most notably heart disease. Finally, the New Guinea natives were completely free of diabetes after 777 of these people were given glucose tolerance tests. It was also found that their blood pressure and cholesterol levels decreased as they got older, instead of increasing as compared to the U.S.

So what is the secret of Optimum Health? The key factor in each of these cultures is that they are eating a high complex carbohydrate, high fiber diet, naturally low in fat and cholesterol, and adequate in plant protein foods. They lead an active life that provides sufficient exercise. They walk or run because there is little modern transportation. In addition, exercise and nutrition help these people to deal with stress more effectively since they are physically fit.

For example, in Hunza the people consume a nutritious 1900 calorie diet consisting of 50 grams of protein. This is less than 14% of total calories from protein, 36 grams of fat (16% of total calories), and over 254 grams of complex carbohydrates (70% of total calories). Their food intake includes chapatis, a whole grain buckwheat pancake, which is a dominant part of their diet, along with large quantities of vegetables such as tomatoes, cucumbers, cabbage, beans, cornmeal and green onion, which are all eaten raw or cooked over a low fire. Also, a variety of fruits are eaten either fresh or dried. Meat, beef, chicken or goat is eaten only a few times per year. The Hunzas do eat cheese or buttermilk daily, but they are very low in fat content (similar to dry curd - only 1 1/2 % fat). The New Guinea natives and the Tarahumaras of Mexico avoid dairy products.

To achieve Optimum Health we recommend you begin a nutritious diet of 20% fat or less, with 10-15% protein (mainly protein found in grains like whole wheat, brown rice, millet and oatmeal) and 60-80% complex carbohydrates (grains, vegies, fruit and beans). Start exercising regularly.

FOOD SUBSTITUTIONS

Simple food substitutions to reduce fat and cholesterol in the diet.
Choose the item with the *.

FOOD	FAT	CHOLESTEROL	CALORIES	% FAT = G. FAT X 9 CAL./T.CAL
Kraft Reduced	0 g.	0 mg.	15	0
Pritikin Italian*	0 g.	0 mg.	6	0
Kraft Regular	8.00 g.	0 mg.	74	97
Mayonnaise, 1 Tbs.	11.00 g.	10 mg.	100	99
Mustard, 1 Tbs.	1.00 g.	0 mg.	15	60
A-1 Sauce*	0 g.	0 mg.	12	0
Whole Milk	8.00 g.	29 mg.	159	56
Lowfat Milk	5.00 g.	14 mg.	121	37
Lite- Milk*, Soy	.40 g.	0 mg.	86	4
Cheddar Cheese 1 oz.	9.40 g.	30 mg.	112	76
Liteline* 1 oz.	2.00 g.	10 mg.	50	36
Egg Yolk	5.70 g.	312 mg.	59	87
Egg White*	0 g.	0 mg.	17	0
Pound Cake	9.00 g.	0 mg.	142	57
Angel Food Cake*	.10 g.	0 mg.	17	1
Avocado	33.00 g.	0 mg.	334	89
Split pea dip*	2.50 g.	0 mg.	145	16
Club Steak	33.00 g.	65 mg.	360	83
Flank Steak*	6.50 g.	64 mg.	163	36
Halibut*	1.00 g.	51 mg.	110	8
Salmon	15.00 g.	68 mg.	250	54
Chicken Breast*	4.50 g.	60 mg.	98	41
Ham, Fat Reduced*	5.00 g.	60 mg.	175	26
Sausage*	40.00 g.	80 mg.	445	81
Bacon	78.00 g.	250 mg.	754	93
Vegetable Oil, 1 Tbs.	14.00 g.	0 mg.	120	100
Butter, 1 Tbs.	12.00 g.	35 mg.	102	98
French Fries	6.60 g.	0 mg.	137	43
Baked Potato*	.05 g.	0 mg.	28	2

*By making simple food substitutions using the items with the *, you would eliminate 572 mg. of cholesterol intake per day, or about 1/2 lb. of clogging cholesterol per year! You would also reduce your daily fat intake by 130 g. (1,100 calories), and your yearly fat intake by 107 lbs.

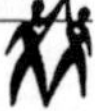

CHAPTER SIX

HOW TO MAINTAIN OR GAIN WEIGHT

MAINTAIN:

After following the Delgado Plan for a time, many people have a tendency to continue to drop below their ideal weight. This may occur because of a subconscious selection and a preference for the low calorie foods like salads, vegetables and soups. The permitted foods like medium calorie fruits and potatoes, and the high calorie grains and legumes become neglected.

When trying to lose weight, most meals should include large amounts of the low and medium calorie foods. After reaching your goal weight, however, these lower calorie foods need to be reduced. **Salads** should be **limited** to **one** small portion a **day**, **vegetables** to **two** small portions a **day**, and **soups** to **three** times a **week** or **eliminated entirely**. Also, **wheat bran** should be **omitted** and **whole grains** or **whole grain foods**, such as **bread should be eaten at every meal** and as **in-between snacks**. In summary to stop losing weight: Remember, the highest calorie foods: oils, margarine, meats, cheese, eggs and sugar have no fiber and cause the fastest weight gain. However, we will not include these foods in a discussion of weight control, since they should not be included as a major part of anyone's diet.

HOW TO MAINTAIN OR GAIN WEIGHT

In practice, for a weight maintenance diet, your daily menu might include a balance between the low calorie vegies, fruit and these high calorie foods:

Breakfast grains - uncooked cereals, museli, granola, nutty rice, pancakes, whole wheat breads.

Lunch grains and high calorie vegetables - Manna or Essene sprouted bread, brown rice, corn, peas, legumes and whole wheat breads with cooked sweet potato spread.

Dinner grains - whole grain entree such as whole wheat spaghetti, corn tortilla enchilada casserole with legumes and cut corn, whole wheat breads.

Snack grains - whole grain breads, Nuggets by NutriGrain, Nutty Rice and raw oatmeal with unsweetened pineapple and other homemade granola.

GAIN:

To gain weight use mostly grains, legumes, breads and pastas, while limiting fruits and vegetables. The maximum calorie intake (3,000 to 4,500) can be consumed each day, concentrating most heavily on the high calorie foods (legumes and grains).

HOW TO MAINTAIN OR GAIN WEIGHT

The following is a typical menu during a weight-gain program:

6:00 a.m. - 2 slices of whole wheat toast, 1/2 grapefruit.

7:30 a.m. - Large bowl of granola, Nuggets cereal (combined with raw oatmeal and Nutri-Grain corn flakes), whole wheat toast.

10:00 a.m. - Bowl of uncooked cereal or whole wheat bread with unsweetened apple butter spread, snack of last night's whole wheat spaghetti.

12:30 p.m. - Brown rice covered with cooked beans, small raw vegetable dish, whole wheat bread.

2:30 p.m. - Whole wheat pita bread stuffed with legumes and brown rice, hummus mixture.

6:00 p.m. - Corn tortilla casserole, small serving of raw vegies, corn, peas and brown rice.

10:00 p.m. - Ear of corn on the cob, multi-grain, sprouted Manna or Essene bread with apple butter.

HOW TO MAINTAIN OR GAIN WEIGHT

For maximum weight gain, muscular growth and strength do the following:

1) Workout at least two to three times a day, six days a week.

2) For weight maintenance workout at least three times a week.

3) Use heavy weights eight to twelve repetitions.

4) Repetitions should be fast and controlled with minimal momentum.

5) Complete each set to the point of "failure" (where you can barely lift the weight on the last repetition).

6) Do one to five exercises per body part.

7) Do one to five sets per exercise.

8) Work on three to four body parts per session.

9) Additional sleep will be needed with daily exercise. You should be able to wake without an alarm if not, go to sleep earlier at night, and add a midday nap if necessary.

10) Do daily aerobic exercise of at least 20 to 30 minutes per session at a "conversation" pace.

11) Eat more complex carbohydrates high in food density like: grains, breads, rice, pasta, beans and yams.

For more detailed information about gaining lean weight read Nick Delgado's Book Mastering the Powers of Your Inner Health.

CHAPTER SEVEN

OSTEOPOROSIS

Osteoporosis is the loss of minerals from the bones, leaving them porous and susceptible to fracture and disability. One billion dollars a year is spent on hip fractures related to bone loss.

Women are eight times more likely to develop a severe case of osteoporosis than men, and more women die each year from osteoporotic fractures than from breast cancer. Estrogen therapy can only slow the loss of bone for about eight years. Estrogen therapy does not cause replacement of lost bone. We have a much better, safer approach.

Exercise and a reduced protein diet are the most effective ways to reabsorb lost bone material. Recent studies reported women 50 to 80 years of age can increase their bone mass 2-3% per year through brisk walking, light weight-lifting or other aerobic movements done at least 30 minutes, 3 to 4 times per week. In ten years you could reabsorb the 30% bone loss that usually disables women by age 75.

The Delgado Diet reduces the protein of the average American diet from over 100 grams down to an ideal intake of between 45 and 80 grams per day. As you consume less protein, you will prevent acid waste products from protein-amino acid digestion. This is the key to stopping osteoporosis, because your body must maintain a Ph balance of 7.2 to 7.4 or you would die. If the blood becomes too acidic (less than 7.2), your bones release calcium into the blood-stream to neutralize the acid. Calcium and other bone minerals like magnesium and zinc serve as a buffer. These minerals act as positive ions to offset the negative ions from acidic blood caused by excess dietary proteins (amino acids).

By consuming far less protein, there will be no acid build-up in the bloodstream. You will stop losing calcium, magnesium and zinc minerals out of the bones. In this way, the Delgado Diet will prevent osteoporosis. This is wonderful news for people who want to avoid hip fractures, spinal column degeneration and loss of teeth, which is so common in the American culture.

The Eskimos of Alaska eat more meat and protein than most Americans. Their diet is 25% protein, the highest in the world. They experience up to 40% greater bone loss by the age of 40 than we do. The Eskimos surpass our calcium intake because they eat the bones of the fish they catch (over 2,000 mg. of calcium per day!) Yet, this concentrated intake of calcium is not enough to prevent osteoporosis. A negative mineral imbalance (more calcium loss out of the bones than is taken in) is caused by their excessive protein intake. Unfortunately, many Americans are mistakenly trying to eat more high protein foods like chicken, fish, nonfat milk, egg whites and protein powders (found in weight loss drinks and body building formulas).

Other studies show elderly vegetarians who eat the proper amount of protein (40 to 90 grams per day) typically have stronger bones and teeth than meat eaters (as determined by X-rays).

The Bantu women of Africa eat only 350 mg. of calcium per day, and give birth to an average of nine children, nursing each child an average of two years (18 years of lactation!). Yet, they have stronger bones and they don't lose their teeth like we do here in the United States. Their children grow up free of dental decay and have excellent bone density. The adults are free of osteoporosis, rickets and they heal well if a fracture should occur (as reported by Walker, Amer. J. Clin. Nutri. 25:518, 1972).

What is their secret? They eat a high complex carbohydrate diet of grains, vegetables and fruit with an adequate amount of protein at 10% (low compared to standards set by dairy industry officials in the U.S.). The Bantus never drink milk or use dairy products after they are weaned at age two.

Ironically, if you use dairy products often to obtain calcium as you get older, you will be getting too much protein and probably will lose more calcium than usual. I avoid most all dairy products because I'm allergic to them (symptoms include diarrhea, fatigue, bloating of stomach from the inability to digest milk - it rots and ferments that can cause mental confusion and disorientation).

Severe to mild symptoms affect many races as they get older. This is only with cow's or goat's milk; human milk would not cause a reaction. Unfortunately, human milk is not available at the store. However, even infants have been allergic to mother's milk if the mother is drinking cow's milk, which seems to pass on to the baby. The mother must stop drinking milk, according to Dr. Lendon Smith, pediatrician, and Dr. Paul Fliess, authorities on breast feeding.

You will get more than enough calcium from corn tortillas, beans, broccoli and cabbage, etc. without the need for dairy products or supplements. (You may take a supplement for calcium provided you also take an equal amount of magnesium). Recent studies by Dr. Anderson monitored people eating high fiber (with phytates) and found no effect (20 to 50 months) on mineral absorption. Levels of calcium, iron, zinc, etc., decrease slightly the first few weeks on the diet, and then stabilize as reported in Diabetes Care (Vol. 3, No. 1 Jan.- Feb. 1980).

To stop osteoporosis switch to the Delgado Health Plan, exercise and quit smoking (just three cigarettes will draw calcium from the bones and start to deposit it into the arteries).

MEAT & POULTRY

Contains NO Carbohydrates

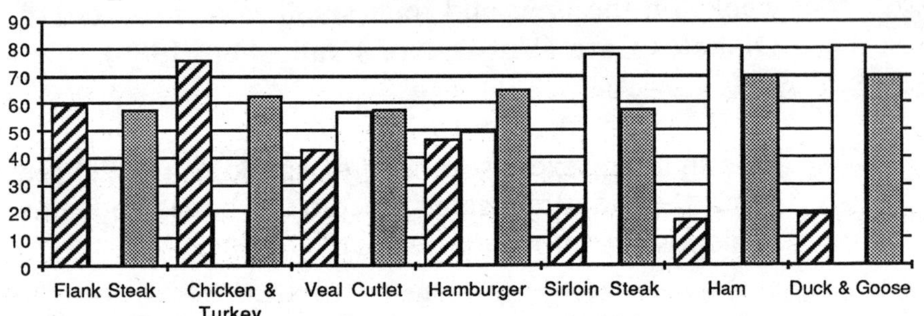

You must avoid eating these high protein: poultry, fish, shellfish, and meats to have strong bones. Also, notice that chicken and fish have just as much cholesterol as stea Cholesterol cloggs your arteries, and excess protein weakens your bones!

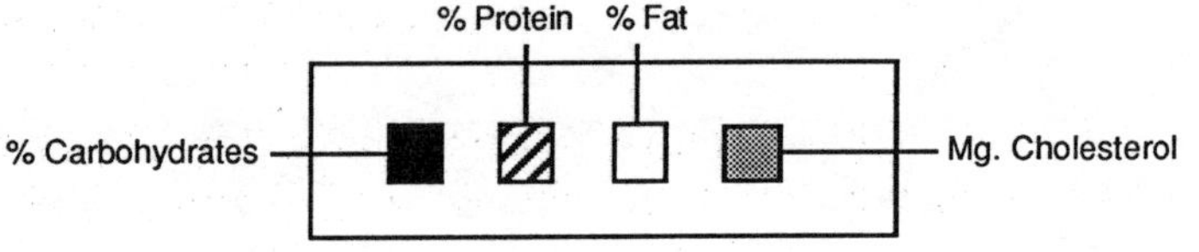

CHOLESTEROL IN 3 1/2 oz. (100 grams) of food (Shown in mg.)

FISH & SHELLFISH

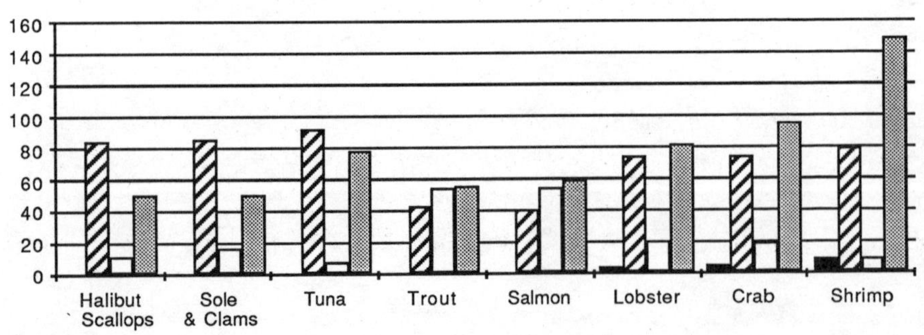

CHAPTER EIGHT

BLOOD PRESSURE AND HYPERTENSION

Over fifty million Americans have high blood pressure (also known as hypertension) and it threatens the lives of one out of every four adults and children. We at Delgado Medical feel like Paul Revere, trying to awaken a sleeping public and alert them to a grave danger. Our message doesn't always reach receptive ears, especially when most doctors and patients depend on drugs to cover up symptoms instead of using diet and exercise to treat the cause.

A normal blood pressure is usually 110/70. That is only the measure of pressure exerted on the artery lining. For example, every time the heart beats, the blood going from the heart through the arteries will exert 110 millimeters of mercury of pressure; that is, it could raise a column of mercury to that height. Between beats there is a pressure exerted by the arteries to return the blood to the heart, and around 70 is considered normal. As pressure is gradually released from this cuff, the doctor can monitor the pressure and pick it up with a stethoscope. The top number (110) is determined by the point where the sound is heard. The second number (70) will show when the beating sound stops under the stethoscope. We have found lower blood pressure, 110/70 or 110/60, is now considered better than 120/80. The chances of heart attacks are double at a diastolic pressure over 80!

One of the main concerns is most people who have high blood pressure will not seek treatment. Many people never even know they have high blood pressure. Why? Because there are no symtoms. It doesn't hurt. You really don't know you have high blood pressure until a doctor or health professional examines your pressure.

Think of high blood pressure as a disease that involves the whole body, not just as something that has gone wrong with the pressure. If your blood pressure is higher, such as 140/90, then we become very concerned. If you maintain a high blood pressure level over ten or twenty years, the arteries begin to become affected. It accelerates deterioration of your arteries, which can leave you susceptible to arterial blowout, possibly a stroke or an aneurysm.

Of course, these can all be very dangerous. Dr. Albert Einstein had an abdominal aneurysm and every time his heart would beat, the weakened point in the artery lining would bulge out. Just as on a basketball, if there is a weakened point, a bubble will form. Unfortunately, one day that abdominal aneurysm burst and Dr. Einstein died. Another problem with high blood pressure is it affects the main target organs: the brain, kidneys and possibly the liver. These organs can become damaged from continual high pressure.

Another name for high blood pressure is hypertension. This name often misleads people, and they believe most cases of high blood pressure are due to tension or being upset. The reality is high blood pressure is related to the thickness of the blood, or the total volume of blood.

If we examine various cultures throughout the world, we find groups of people who eat large amounts of salt have an alarming rate of high blood pressure. For example, 40% of the population in northern Japan eat from 18 to 30 grams of salt daily, have high blood pressure and one of the highest death rates from stroke (arterial blowout) in the world. If we compare this Japanese culture to the New Guinea natives who eat a low-salt diet and low-fat diet, we find they have no incidence of high blood pressure, and even when they reach age 60, they still have a 110/60 blood pressure.

What is it about salt that increases the blood pressure? Salt causes fluid retention. If you use salt in your foods, this excess salt will absorb fluid into your bloodstream, adding 5-7 extra pounds of water weight to your bloodstream. This extra weight will create more pressure every time your heart beats. For example, when you turn on the garden hose and force more fluid through it, the pressure goes up.

We know high blood pressure is not hereditary. Studies were done on Japanese who migrated to other countries where they eat less salt, and their blood pressure began to drop down. In another study of high school students in Japan, one group was taught how to lower salt in the diet. Another group, the control group, continued eating as much salt as they wanted. At the end of the study, the group who ate the most salt had somewhat higher blood pressure. The group who kept their salt intake down maintained a normal blood pressure.

In a 1975 study, Dr. Iacono of the Agricultural Department instructed a group of people who were eating 10 grams of salt per day (the average American intake) to continue eating the same amount of salt while cutting back on the amount of fat in their diet. Instead of eating the usual 35-43% fat diet, he showed them how to reduce their fat intake to under 25% fat. They switched to nonfat milk instead of whole milk, chicken, fish and turkey instead of red, fatty meats. They cut back on the use of butter, margarine and oils, and started steaming and broiling their foods.

Within ten days, these patients lowered their blood pressure a full 10%, both the systolic and diastolic numbers. When they started eating the same high fat diet as before, their blood pressure rose. Dr. Iacono had discovered the amount of fat in the diet affected blood pressure far more than the amount of salt.

Don't misunderstand - we're suggesting you do reduce the salt in your diet, but once you reduce the salt, the far greater cause of high blood pressure is fat in the diet.

If you reduce salt in the diet and your blood pressure doesn't come down to normal, you have to search for other possible causes. If a doctor examines you, and cannot find the problem, you may be told you have "essential hypertension," which means "of unknown cause." At this point, you may be given medications to control your blood pressure.

But, medications are no longer considered a safe form of treatment. 35% of those on these medications must stop taking them because of serious side effects. Diuretics may double your chances of sudden death due to heart failure. These drugs raise your blood cholesterol, triglycerides and glucose. Sir William Osler, a famous physician, stated, "One of the first duties of the physician is to educate the masses not to take medicine." Benjamin Franklin said, "It is the best physician that knows the worthlessness of most medicines." If you are on medications now, there is a safer, more effective solution.

If you follow our natural approach to lowering blood pressure, you'll be much safer than depending on medications for the rest of your life. Prolonged use of these medications can cause kidney damage and high urea nitrogen levels, which can cause kidney failure. You may develop gouty arthritis because uric acid levels elevate from certain blood pressure medications. These drugs also can cause elevation of the blood glucose level and you could become diabetic. Surprisingly, male impotency can result as a side effect from blood pressure medications.

Research studies showed over 50% of the men tested became sexually impotent because the blood flow was reduced so much from the blood pressure medications they were unable to maintain an erection. These drugs have also reported to cause apathy and diminished sexual excitability. The brain function is altered by blood pressure beta-blocker drugs, and reports of failing memory, headaches, dizziness, drowsiness, depression, nightmares and a decline in intellectual power have been noted as side effects.

According to Dr. Cleaves Bennett, M.D., hypertension specialist, there are four major types of medication that are currently used in the treatment of high blood pressure: the diuretics, the blockers, the vasodilators and the inhibitors.

1) The best the diuretics can do is rid your body of some salt. You could do that by cutting down on the amount of salt you eat. Diuretics often don't work if they're not used correctly and if they don't work it is harder for the other drugs to work as well. A good diet would do what diuretics do - and do it better.

2) The blockers leave you drowsy when they work, and when they don't make you drowsy, they can't control your blood pressure in a routine domestic crisis or a traffic jam. Stress management would do what the blockers do much better.

3) The vasodilators diminish the pressure in the blood vessels by acting directly on the muscles of the arterioles. A lowfat diet and salt reduction would do a better job of controlling the fluid content of the blood vessels, and stress management with exercise would relax the muscles in the arterioles more effectively.

4) The endocrine inhibitors: Captopril is a drug that blocks the formation of angiotensin, a hormone that can raise the blood pressure profoundly. This overactive renin-angiotensin problem rarely occurs. However, when it does it is usually caused by cholesterol blockages of the arteries leading to the kidneys. The drug Captopril only works for a while, until the body learns to counteract the effect of the drug by making more of the hormone. The best solution is the unclog the arteries to the kidneys by the Delgado Zero Cholesterol Diet. It may take two or three years, but diet does get to the cause of the problem instead of covering it up with drugs.

Many patients assume the medications they take must be good for them because their blood pressure is lower. It simply isn't true. The Journal of the American Medical Association published a recent report entitled, "Multiple Risk Factor Intervention Trial (1982). The authors described their results as "ambiguous but disquieting." They found the use of pharmacologic therapy -drugs-in the treatment of some hypertensives seems associated with "an increased coronary heart disease mortality." In simple English, they found that taking a diuretic for high blood pressure might lower the blood pressure while raising the total risk of dying from heart disease.

Unfortunately, most doctors can't possibly read all the articles in all the medical journals. A study published in the American Journal of Medicine (1982) showed many doctors are more influenced by the glossy color handouts drug salesmen pass around than they are by articles in the medical journals. Drug companies make their advertising literature much easier to read than the journals, with their small print and extensive footnotes.

As a result, research that encourages the use of drugs is often more familiar to doctors. After all, no one goes from doctor to doctor promoting because if you take care of yourself through diet and exercise, you may not need any drugs. That approach won't sell anything. I assure you that for every drug there is a company representative knocking on the doctors' doors showing beautiful brochures with data to support the drugs' use. If the representative can sell your doctor on a drug, then the doctor can sell hundreds of patients on it and there are huge profits to be made.

The first week you start our program, you should see one of our doctors or your doctor. Under a doctors supervision, you will need to decrease slowly, day by day, the dosage you're taking now and monitor your blood pressure. Generally, you should begin reducing or stopping the strongest first, the one that causes the worst side effects. Usually, the strongest medications are the ones a doctor adds last. Here is a list showing an order in which medications can be dealt with; those in Step 1 are the most powerful.

STEP-DOWN MEDICATIONS

Step 1: Minoxidil, guanethidine.

Step 2: Hydralazine, captopril, clonidine, prazosin, methyldopa, reserpine.

Step 3: Beta Blockers (propanolol, metoprolol, nadolol, atenolol): reduce dosage slowly, usually cut in half every three days.

Step 4: Diuretics (furosemide, hydrochlorothiazide, other thiazides, ethacrynic acid, spironolactone, triamterene, amiloride).

Step 5: Off all medications.

Proceed under your doctors supervision, while monitoring your blood pressure in the doctors office and at home. Begin with the most powerful drugs in Step 1 and work through to Step 5. When the dosage is large, cutting the amount of one type of medications by a third or half may be the first step.

Wait about three days before beginning the next decrease in dosage of this medication. When you have reached the smallest dosage in which the medication is packaged, then the next step is to stop it altogether. If with the dietary change, blood pressure falls to levels that are too low to be on medications, such as 110/70 or lower, or if a person becomes dizzy, then the dosages should be lowered more rapidly. When adjusting medications in this manner, try to keep the blood pressure below 160/100. Don't worry if the pressure is this high for a few days. This elevation for a short time does not place you in any extra danger.

However, most people with high blood pressure have a very serious disease of the arteries and therefore are at a high risk of having a hazardous complication. Even so, if a stroke or heart attack did occur while an individual was making adjustments, often it would be a coincidence. The actual cause of these events would be many years of serious damage to the arteries from abuses caused by diet and lifestyle, not from the reduction in medication and the slight rise in blood pressure which sometimes follows a lower dosage.

Actually, during this short period of adjustment, the danger is greater from too much medication than too little. Over-enthusiastic treatment of blood pressure can be dangerous. The attempt to lower blood pressure to normal levels with medication in patients with extensive atherosclerosis has been shown to result in a fivefold increase in heart attacks.

Beta blockers should be reduced slowly, because rapid withdrawal can cause bothersome strong or rapid heartbeats. There is also some evidence that too rapid a decrease in dosage of beta blockers will cause chest pains and heart attacks in susceptible patients. On the other hand, withdrawal of some medications, such as clonidine, may cause a rapid rise in blood pressure, with symtoms of nervousness, agitation and headache. The medication should be reduced slowly, at intervals of three days.

Your goal is to lower your blood pressure to 110/70 or less without medication. Some people will not reach this ideal pressure, even following a strict low-salt, low-fat vegetarian diet and clean lifestyle, because the damage to the circulatory system is already too severe. Also, a small minority of people have hypertension from causes other than years of poor diet and lifestyle practices, which need attention other than changes in their habits. A doctor will need to identify these rare cases.

If we examine people on a high fat diet and look at their bloodstream, the red blood cells are stuck together. Fat, whether animal or vegetable in origin, will cause the blood cells to stick together and thicken the blood. This forces the blood pressure to go up, because the cells can barely get through the smaller blood vessels, the capillaries. When you start on the Delgado Plan and exercise 30 minutes or more per day, the red blood cells become evenly separated rapidly. Your blood pressure will start to come down almost immediately.

I'd like to summarize the best ways to lower blood pressure. The first and most important step is to reduce fat in your diet and start eating more complex carbohydrates. The second would be to cut back on your salt use. Instead of salt on your foods and in cooking, use onion powder, garlic powder, cayenne pepper and other spices. Step three is lose weight. If you're overweight, the body has to work harder to maintain blood flow.

Another way to lower blood pressure is through aerobic exercise, such as brisk walking, jogging or using mini-trampolines. We have found aerobic exercising for one-half to an hour per day, will help to reduce the fat levels in your bloodstream and dilate blood vessels. Studies show for most people, blood pressure will come down dramatically within seven weeks. Recent studies show caffeine in soda drinks or coffee, nicotine in cigarettes, and alcohol will promote high blood pressure.

We have also found reducing cholesterol intake in the diet may help to reduce blood pressure significantly. Cholesterol reduction is important because if your arteries are loaded with plaques, it will be more difficult for the blood to flow through the clogged arteries. Reducing cholesterol then, is one of your goals, and it also can help to prevent aneurysms and the weakening of the artery linings.

Reduction of stress is also important, although continued stress is not the main cause of high blood pressure. It may temporarily elevate your blood pressure while you're upset, but stress cannot maintain it chronically day after day, year after year. If your blood pressure is elevated, you need to improve the blood flow first and then start working toward reducing stress.

You'll need to see one of our doctors to reduce medications as needed. When you start following these points, you're blood pressure will come down rapidly, almost dramatically. If you do not reduce blood pressure medications, you may have too low of a blood pressure because our plan is so powerful! One possible symptom of too low blood pressure would be to become weak or dizzy when you try to get up after sitting.

BLOOD PRESSURE AND HYPERTENSION

At Delgado Medical we have one of the highest success rates in the country helping people to control blood pressure. If you come to our clinic we can examine your eating habits and health profile. In this way we can establish the course of treatment for people who have high blood pressure. Call us for details.

SODIUM

IN PROCESSED FOODS		IN FRESH & LOW SODIUM FOODS	
Arby's Ham & Cheese (8 oz.)	1,745 mg.	Homemade sandwich - whole wheat, chicken, tomato, lettuce (9 oz.)	215 mg.
Jumbo Jack Hamburger (9 oz.)	1,665 mg.		
Weight Watchers Oriental Chicken (12 oz.)	1,595 mg.	Pritikin Chicken Broth (12 oz.)	150 mg.
Flour, self-rising (cup)	1,349 mg.	Flour, Whole Wheat (cup)	2 mg.
Kentucky Fried Chicken (12 oz.)	1,500 mg.	Chicken breast, baked (12 oz.)	225 mg.
Oscar Mayer Wieners (3.2 oz.)	1,028 mg.		
McDonald's Big Mac (7.2 oz.)	1,010 mg.	Kasha hamburger, whole wheat (7 oz.)	250 mg.
Burger King Whopper (9 oz.)	1,000 mg.		
Country Hearth white bread (2 slices)	1,000 mg.	Pritikin-Whole Wheat, Rye, Multi-Grain (2 slices):	210 mg.
Sauerkraut (1/2 cup)	878 mg.	Cabbage (1/2 cup)	7 mg.
Pizza, Cheese (2 slices, 5.5 oz.)	800 mg.	Pizza, Whole Wheat, vegies, no cheese (2 slices)	70 mg.
Gerber Beef & Egg Noodles baby food (jar)	705 mg.	Baby food vegies (jar)	
Kraft Processed Cheese (1.5 oz.)	698 mg.	Ricotta, part skim cheese (1.5 oz.)	58 mg.
Minute Rice Long Grain white (1/2 cup)	570 mg.	Brown rice (1/2 cup)	1 mg.
Tomato Paste with salt (1/2 cup)	524 mg.	Tomato Paste without salt (1/2 cup)	50 mg.
Carnation Slender Diet drink (1/2 cup)	500 mg.	Mineral water & pineapple juice (1/2 c.)	15mg.
Flour Tortillas (1)	473 mg.	Corn Tortillas (1)	26 mg.
Tomato juice, regular (1/2 cup)	437 mg.	Tomato juice, low sodium (1/2 cup)	4 mg.
Soy sauce, regular (tsp.)	358 mg.	Soy sauce, salt-reduced Kikkoman (tsp)	182 mg.
Cheddar Cheese (1.5 oz.)	340 mg.	Ricotta, park skim (1.5 oz.)	58 mg.
Whole canned tomatoes, drained (1/2 cup)	337 mg.	Tomatoes, fresh (1/2 cup)	4 mg.
Campbell's Vegetable soup (7 oz.)	700 mg.	Pritikin vegetable soup (7 oz.)	150 mg.
Campbell's Chicken Noodles (7 oz.)	900 mg.	Prit. chicken soup, Ribbon Pasta (7 oz.)	17 mg.
Del Monte Tomato Sauce (1/2 cup)	700 mg.	Pritikin tomato soup & pieces (1/2 c.)	65 mg.
Canned vegetables, drained			
Asparagus (1/2 cup)	280 mg.	Asparagus (1/2 cup)	1 mg.
Lima beans (1/2 cup)	200 mg.	Lima beans (1/2 cup)	1 mg.
Peas (1/2 cup)	200 mg.	Peas (1/2 cup)	1 mg.
Beets (1/2 cup)	195 mg.	Beets (1/2 cup)	40 mg.
Tomato puree (1/2 cup)	249 mg.	Tomatoes, blended fresh (1/2 cup)	4 mg.
Capers (tbsp.)	233 mg.	Enrico's mild salsa, no salt (tbsp.)	1 mg.
Mild chili salsa (tbsp.)	175 mg.	Pritikin Mexican Sauce (2 oz.)	17 mg.
French Fries (5 oz.)	220 mg.	Potatoes, sliced, baked crisp (5 oz.)	2 mg.
Ragu Spaghetti Sauce (4 oz.)	640 mg.	Pritikin or Johnson's sauce (4 oz.)	35 mg.
Kraft Italian oil-free (tbsp.)	210 mg.	Pritikin Italian salad dressing (tbsp.)	0 mg.
		El Molino Italian oil-free (tbsp.)	40 mg.
Kraft French dressing (tbsp.)	125 mg.	Pritikin Italian salad dressing (tbsp.)	0 mg.
Mustard, prepared (tsp.)	63 mg.	Hain Mustard, unsalted (tsp.)	3 mg.
Ketchup, Del Monte (tbsp.)	169 mg.	Ketchup, Del Monte, no salt (tbsp.)	5 mg.
Quaker Instant Oatmeal (3/4 cup)	252 mg.	Quaker Old Fashioned Rolled Oats, ckd (3/4 cup)	1 mg.

The total intake of sodium for most individuals should be about 2,000 mg. (or less) per day. All foods naturally contain some sodium, so that if none of these high sodium foods on the processed food column were consumed, a person would take in about 400 - 2,000 mg. per day. If a product contains less than 175 mg. of sodium per serving, consider it "safe." Fresh foods are much lower in sodium. Low sodium foods are good only if they don't have added fat and sugar. For example, Campbells's low sodium tomato soup is too high in fat, sugar and cholesterol, and Campbells's regular tomato soup is too high in sodium, so use the Pritikin tomato soup instead. Also, Health Valley soups are low enough in sodium and fat and they are tasty.

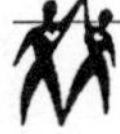

CHAPTER NINE

STRESS

A problem that we all face in our fast-paced society is stress. Stress does not directly cause high blood pressure. For example, you're upset, you have a fight with a loved one - spouse, boyfriend, girlfriend, etc. and what happens? Perhaps you neglect yourself, you don't exercise or you eat all the wrong foods. You might get the nervous nibbles and start eating compulsively. Stress has a very powerful effect on our lives and how we live. I'd like to share with you ways to reduce stress and get control of your life.

Are you a Type A personality? Are you under a great deal of stress? For instance, do you rush your speech? Do you hurry other people's speech? Do you hurry when you eat? Do you never seem to catch up? Do you schedule more activities than you have time to complete? Do you often try to do several things at once? Notice how often you'll be driving on the freeway and see other drivers shaving, drinking coffee and reading at the same time!

Do you drive fast most of the time? Most of us are in such a hurry, instead of scheduling enough time to get to our destination. This can be very upsetting, especially when you become impatient if others are driving too slow. Do you have an intense drive, a constant struggle to get ahead? Do you detest wasting time and race with the clock, constantly looking at your watch? Of course, having an intense drive, struggling to get ahead and watching your time is all part of an executive's lifestyle. However, you can still be in control without the damaging effects of stress.

Do you have little time for relaxation, intimacy or enjoying your environment? In other words, do you set aside time to go to the movies, the beach, admire a sunset? You need to schedule time for activities you really enjoy. Some people have a difficult time thinking of things they like to do. Do you compete with others to get ahead and have trouble returning to normal after intense stress? These are some important areas to consider because if stress is affecting your health and the way you function, then you have a major problem.

When we are under stress, we all react the same way with what we call the "fight or flight" syndrome. Your brain will immediately relay a signal and release certain hormones, including ACTH and adrenaline, if you become upset or perceive stress. These hormones enter the bloodstream and cause rapid physiological changes. You breathe faster, your heart beats faster, your blood sugar levels increase and the digestive tract slows down. The muscles in your hands and feet tighten up. Your hands get cold because your blood vessels are constricting. Your blood pressure goes up while you're under stress, your eyes dilate and your hair stands on end.

In primitive times this type of reaction was to your benefit. If you had to run or fight to save your life, you could meet the demands with this excess intensity, energy and concentration. But, let's imagine you're driving on the freeway and someone cuts in front of you. You grab the steering wheel, you honk the horn and you yell at the other driver. You get so upset and you go through those stress responses. Several hours later, the bloodstream is fired up with adrenaline and this can cause you considerable problems.

Stress can cause an increase in stomach acids that are secreted in the abdominal area. If there is no fibrous food present in the stomach, the acids begin to eat away at the stomach lining, which is the principal cause of ulcers. We have also found stress-related ulcers can be reduced significantly if we stay in control of the situation.

To protect yourself from ulcers, you must also follow a high fiber protective diet. A bland diet, devoid of fiber used to be the recommended plan to follow if you had ulcers. We now know that diets lacking fiber will increase the development rate of ulcers.

In a study conducted during World War II, groups of officers, safe behind enemy lines, were examined and found to have a high rate of ulcers. These men were eating processed foods, white bread, eggs, butter, cheese, etc., all foods containing no fiber. This was very surprising because the men on the front lines who were shot at, in a life threatening situation and who were under a great deal more stress, had no ulcers. Why? The men on the front lines were only served basic staples - whole oatmeal, whole brown rice, whole wheat bread, potatoes, etc. They had none of the processed, sugary, salty foods available only to the officers.

Based on this evidence, a high fiber diet will help to reduce the ulcer significantly, usually within a period of two years. To increase your fiber intake, eat beans, peas, yams, raw carrots and purnes. All of these foods are rich in soothing fiber. You can use additional wheat bran in your whole grain cereals. Eat large amounts of brown rice and whole oatmeal.

What is it about fiber that protects you from ulcers? We have found eating frequent meals (5-10 meals daily) of high complex carbohydrate fiber food creates an artificial mucus lining in the intestinal tract and in the stomach. Even if the stomach's acids are secreted when you become upset, the artificial mucus lining will protect the stomach lining from being eaten away. This prevents ulcers and bleeding ulcers.

We want to help you reduce stress directly. One of the most effective techniques is called the "Quieting Response." This technique was developed by Dr. Charles Strobel, using bio-feedback equipment. When Dr. Strobel noticed people upset, he'd hook them up to his equipment and teach them how to calm and relax themselves by listening to the machine and monitoring their progress through bio-feedback. Although the equipment was effective, he found it was difficult for people to transfer what they had learned from these machines to their day-to-day environment. Because of this problem, Dr. Strobel developed this very effective technique called the "Quieting Response." You can use it any time during the day, as often as needed, whenever you are under stress.

Here are the steps to the "Quieting Response." First, when you recognize you're under stress, you need to smile immediately. You may not know it, but you can create 250,000 different facial expressions and the smile nuerologically effects the brain and begins to calm you. Earlier, you learned the brain is the first to perceive stress and releases these hormones, so when you smile, you're beginning to gain control. Of course, if you are in an intense situation, such as an argument, and you smile outwardly, you may get punched in the nose! In that situation, it would obviously be better to smile inwardly. It may take a little practice, but it works very well.

The next step is to say to yourself, "I am in control and calm and I can handle this situation." This is very important to keep repeating to yourself.

The third step is to take two slow, easy, deep breaths through your nose. Relax and breathe. Remember, this is all happening in less than six seconds, so you need to create it as an automatic response.

Then, you need to be sure your jaw is loose and relaxed, because if your jaw is tight, it's going to cause stress. Your tongue should be resting on the lower part of your jaw, and your shoulders should be limp and relaxed. Be in control of your body and your mind. Keep repeating to yourself "I am in control."

The final step is to resume the normal activity. Don't dwell on what upset you. Take your mind off the problem and go on. Keep in mind you'll have to practice this technique for a short time until it becomes automatic.

We are excited about a new, effective stress management model using techniques of N.L.P. (Nuerolinguistic programming). the "Stress to Success" approach has been thoroughly tested at two major hospitals in Beverly Hills and Century City. First, the "stressed" patient is placed in a space-age like capsule, sitting in a comfortable chair. Once comfortably seated inside, you become aware that this is your time to rejuvenate and relax, as the lights dim and the computer controlled program begins. For up to thirty minutes, you drift off into a deep state of relaxation and solitude. You are guided by a voice, set against a background of melodic music and natural sounds. Pictures and images are seen in your mind's eye. Shifting patterns of light, color, sound, sensations and aromas are experienced and used in a way to uniquely create positive changes in your behavior. Anxiety and destructive tensions melt away. Your mind eases and your body releases into an optimally vacationed and exhilarating state. You leave refreshed, invigorated and clear-minded. Electrodes monitor changes in your temperature, bodily impulses and heart rate. A printout of the data collected lends proof to this powerful technology.

After four to twelve treatments of fifteen to thirty minutes each, you may experience a 60% increase in energy, 30% increase in relaxation, 58% less stress and a 47% reduction in pain. You also take a cassette tape to play as needed to turn stress to success. the tape will trigger the same calming, powerful effects you experienced inside the sound-proof capsule. It works better than any method we have investigated. Contact us at Delgado Medical for more information.

If you are under stress, you also can be affected by the foods you eat. According to a scientific study reported in Epidemiological Journal, 1978, Volume 107, people were monitored according to their personalities (Type A or B). They found the Type A nervous individuals had a higher death rate from heart disease than the calm, relaxed individual (Type B). As a result, it was assumed the higher death rate was due to the high stress levels involved.

When they decided to check on diet, the scientists were amazed to find the Type A individuals were eating 20% more cholesterol and 10% more saturated fats than the Type B individuals. They "theorized" that possibly it was the food that led to severe heart conditions.

Later, they conducted a follow up study in Framingham, Massachusetts, and to everyone's surprise they were unable to reproduce the same results. This time the Type B personalities had the higher death rate because now they were eating more fat and cholesterol than the Type A person.

Stress can be very harmful for an individual with a heart condition. But, if you follow the Delgado Plan, you'll find when you get upset or stressful that you'll be more in control and feel more relaxed. Your circulation will be better and stress will not affect you so dangerously.

We've examined many people at our Delgado Medical Clinic and I'd like to share with you a typical case, a gentleman who visited us. We'll call him John Smith, age 53 and married. His chief complaint was fatigue. When he'd wake up in the morning he could hardly get himself out of bed. He was always tired and lacked energy. He also had difficulty concentrating and a decrease in sexual energy.

In talking with him, we learned he was a CPA, a very stressful job according to our patient. We've found, though, most professions - doctor, real estate agents, housewives - are all under stress! This patient had been at the same job for 20 years. He worked 10 to 12 hours per day, five to six days a week and he often brought work home with him. We would call this man a "workaholic." Here, though, work itself didn't seem to be the cause of stress. We checked further to find what could be causing his complaints.

When this patient would become upset or find himself under a great deal of stress, he would use medications such as valium to calm his nerves. Valium is now considered one of the most commonly used prescription drugs in this country, with sales over $400,000,000. Mr. Smith also used Diazide and Dalmane for his blood pressure.

Our patient also smoked about 40 cigarettes per day, drank a large glass of wine daily and five whiskey cocktails per week. He also drank eight to ten cups of coffee per day.

Mr. Smith exercised only sporadically, and slept only about five to six hours per night. Considering the large amounts of coffee he consumed (about 1,250 milligrams of caffeine), it was surprising he could sleep at all!

He was overweight about 35 pounds and had a "typical" understanding of nutrition. His usual breakfast consisted of toast with butter, coffee, eggs and sausage. For lunch he would eat steak, french fries and pie. Dinner would be more meat, vegetables and dessert. Later, he'd snack on nuts, cheese, potato chips and alcoholic drinks. He used salt on his food, and about 16 teaspoons of sugar with whole milk in his coffee every day. He ate all the wrong foods daily, and rarely ate fruits, vegetables or cereals.

We also learned he ate about six eggs per week. Remember, since the body can only get rid of 100 milligrams of cholesterol per day, he had a severe build-up. His cholesterol level was 420! That is very, very high as you know. It should be 100 plus your age, and never over 160. His triglycerides were 260 because of the fatty foods he was eating.

When questioned about his sexual problems, he said was "just too tired, because I'm 53 years old. What do you expect?" Many people believe as we get older, we're supposed to slow down. Our patient thought it was inevitable that with old age we become decrepit and incapable of living life to the fullest.

Of course, we shared our approach with Mr. Smith and showed him how to reduce the stress in his life. The great news is he reduced his cholesterol and triglyceride levels, lost weight and increased his energy level. Within a short time, his sex life was back to normal, too. As you can see, there are many benefits to eating properly, exercising and reducing stress!

CHAPTER TEN

CANCER: STOMACH, LIVER, LEUKEMIA

Cancer is probably one of the most feared diseases that affects our population. It claims over 400,000 lives each year and one out of four adults will contract cancer and die from this serious disease. It is the second leading cause of death in this country, after atherosclerosis or hardening of the arteries.

We have reviewed information about the causes of cancer and we now know a great deal about how to prevent it. Within the last few years both the National Cancer Institute and the American Cancer Society have published some of the largest documented reports (nearly 600 pages) following the many studies conducted by medical research departments across the country. These reports tell us over 54% of cancers are preventable throught nutritional dietary changes. Unfortunately, there is very little financing to educate the public about nutrition, and most people have not heard about these anti-cancer reports. There is no way for a pharmaceutical company to patent the diet or for any other private groups to gain the finances to pay for newspaper, TV and radio publicity and education for the prevention of cancer. Unless the government sponsors massive education campaigns, it is up to us then, to spread the word and let people know there are several ways to avoid many types of cancer.

First we must understand what cancer is. Cancer is considered a mutation of the cells as they develop and grow. The actual function of the cell is altered in its capability to function as a normal cell. For example, under normal circumstances a liver cell reproduces another liver cell. But, during the production of additional cells, if the cell mutates and loses its ability to function as a viable liver cell, and eventually reproduces repeatedly, a tumor will form. A tumor is a growth or a group of cells that have no proper function in the body. They absorb energy and eat the body alive by replacing the function of essential organs.

While cancer mutations do occur from environmental factors, we are now learning a far greater cause of mutations is the basic oxygen-carrying capacity of the body. Dr. Otto Warburg of Germany, two time Nobel Prize winner, found a relationship between low oxygen levels and cancer. His work was later carried on by Dr. Goldblat, who conducted a series of fascinating experiments dating back to the 1950's. He took cardiac cells from an actual heart, had them reproduced and these heart cells were then put into two separate test tubes. One group of cells was deprived of oxygen while the other group was provided proper oxygen and hemoglobin to maintain its life.

In the group of cells deprived of oxygen, most of the cells died as you would expect. Yet, some cells survived and those surviving cells mutated, or changed their chromosomal makeup. These mutated cells became malignant. During one years time, they injected these cells into animals and all the animals died of cancer. When doctors compared the malignant cells to the same original cardiac cell that received proper oxygen and hemoglobin after a period of two years, they found there were no malignant cells present in the test tube. They injected the cells into animals and no cancers developed. We have found, therefore, oxygen deprivation is a principal cause of mutated cells.

What could cause oxygen deprivation in the human body? We know high fat levels in the diet deprive the body of oxygen, while the low-fat Delgado Plan will increase the amount of oxygen. Another way to fight cancer would be to increase your oxygen levels using exercise. One group of 1,000 long distance runners was found to have only 1/7 the cancer deaths of the general population. We have also discovered through autopsy report when blood vessels are examined, blockages of plaque or clots of cholesterol are present. Downstream of the blockages, where there is not enough oxygen reaching the cells, mutations occur or cancer develops. You need to reduce your cholesterol consumption to reduce the chance of plaques and cancer.

There are several different causes of cancer. If we look throughout the world, we discover stomach cancer, for example, is very high in Japan. But, when the Japanese migrate to the United States, the first generation has a one-third lower stomach cancer rate. Over time they become "Americanized" and adopt the American lifestyle, and eventually the stomach cancer rate is almost non-existent.

What is it about the Japanese diet or lifestyle that causes stomach cancer? We can identify several factors. First, the Japanese pickle their fish to preserve it in sodium nitrates, and we know these can turn into nitrosamines. Since there is a low vitamin C content in the Japanese diet, and nothing to prevent these nitrosamines from forming, we then have potential stomach cancer.

The second, and probably the greatest cause of stomach cancer in the Japanese, is the fact they used white rice coated with talcum powder. Talcum powder is mined in the same place as asbestos. If you can imagine, they used this talcum powder on the rice for cosmetic purposes - it made the rice look whiter. The result is they have had a tremendously higher rate of stomach cancer. Fortunately, the Japanese banned the use of talcum powder in rice by the end of the 1980's. Other forms of rice, brown and Chinese white rice, for example have no talcum powder.

The third factor for the Japanese is their excessive use of salt. They use 20 to 30 grams of salt per day, which may aggravate the stomach lining.

If we examine the Japanese rate of colon cancer, we discover they have a much lower rate of colon cancer per every hundred people. However, those Japanese who migrated from Japan to the United States, develop colon cancer at a rate of two and one-half times greater than their relatives of the same genetic race. If we compare the rate in Japan to the United States population as a whole, we find over four to five times the rate of colon cancer in the U.S. If the Japanese people adopt all the typical U.S. habits and food patterns, they develop colon cancer. Colon cancer, we have discovered is related to dietary factors. It's related to a lack of fiber and an overconsumption of fat in the diet, and we'll discuss that in more detail a little further on.

Pancreatic cancer is also somewhat low in Japan and much higher in the U.S. There is some correlation now with high fat diets and pancreatic cancer.

Leukemia is a cancer in which an overproduction of a certain type of white blood cell crowds out the function of other cells. Leukemia is also much higher in the U.S. In the journal "Science" (Vol. 213, 1981), it was reported more than 20% of the U.S. dairy cows were infected with leukemia viruses. When these viruses were fed to chimpanzees, the experimental animals developed leukemia. Perhaps the fact the U.S. consumes more dairy products than all other nations combined accounts for this higher rate of leukemia in the U.S. There is also some early indication excessive fat levels may lead to many cases of leukemia. While leukemia can be treated with certain types of therapies, once a person develops cancer of any sort, it becomes a very serious situation.

There are several different mutations that can occur from various types of carcinogens. Recently we have discovered smoking food or charbroiling meat, especially higher fat cuts of meat, will increase the rate of carcinogenic property. For example, one pound of smoked mutton or lamb contains the equivalent of 250 cigarettes in carcinogenic properties. A quarter pound of charbroiled hamburger would contain more than a 50 cigarette equivalent. It's very upsetting for me to see certain hamburger chains promote fund raising activities to discover the cause of cancer, and yet children rush to these hamburger stands and potentially increase their risk of cancer dramatically.

The mutations that occur from benzo pyrene are a result of the fat dripping down onto the hot surface underneath and pyrolyzing, or changing chemically, and seeping back into the meat, where it remains. When you eat the meat, you ingest these carcinogenic properties. My suggestion is you prepare your meat differently. For example, when you select lower fat meats, such as chicken, fish or turkey, it's best to cook them in a casserole so the meat isn't in direct contact with a hot surface. If you use other types of cooking processes, such as a microwave, there is an avoidance of this benzo pyrene buildup.

Another cause of cancer that we have identified is related to an aflatoxin, which is a powerful carcinogen that is excreted from a fungus caller Aspergillus flavus. This fungus generally grows on peanuts and other types of foods on occasion. Peanuts, though, are the most significant source. In Mozambique, where most of their diet is composed of peanuts, they have one of the highest rates of liver cancer in the world. You might think it's very unfortunate this poor group of people has such a high rate of liver cancer. Yet, when "Consumer Reports" analyzed over 14 different brands of peanuts and peanut butter, they found conclusively every brand of peanut butter had aflatoxin in it. Just because you eat peanut butter doesn't mean you'll develop liver cancer, since it is dose related. But, after several years of use, you very well could.

One study was done on starving Indian children who had been shipped peanut flour. They unknowingly ate the peanut flour that was contaminated with aflatoxin. It was found just three parts per million of aflatoxin over a 30-day period led to cirrhotic liver and death.

Liver cancer is on the increase in the United States today, and I'm always concerned when children are sent to school with their peanut butter and jelly sandwiches. We suggest you switch to almond butter or cashew butter, or any other kind of nut or seed. Peanuts are not a nut or seed at all, but a legume. They grow underground. All other nuts and seeds grow on top of land on vines or trees, and are rarely found to have fungus.

However, because peanuts do grow underground, they have a moist shell. It absorbs the moisture from the soil, and when it is pulled up from the ground, it's a fertile bed for this fungus, Aspergilus flavus, to grow. Even if you cook the peanuts, roast them, etc., it does not get rid of the aflatoxin. You may kill the fungus, but the aflatoxin is the excretion product, and it remains. Again, we highly recommend you reduce the use of peanuts. Occasionally would be fine, but don't use them regularly. All other nuts and seeds are safer to use, but because of their high fat content, only use them in small quantities -up to two ounces per day.

FATS, OILS & LARD

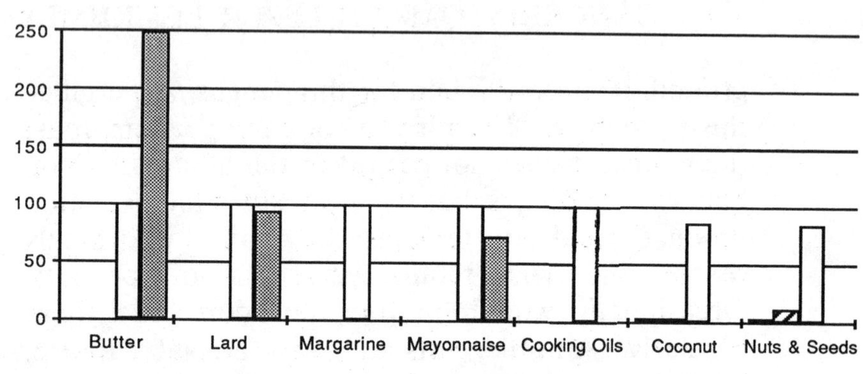

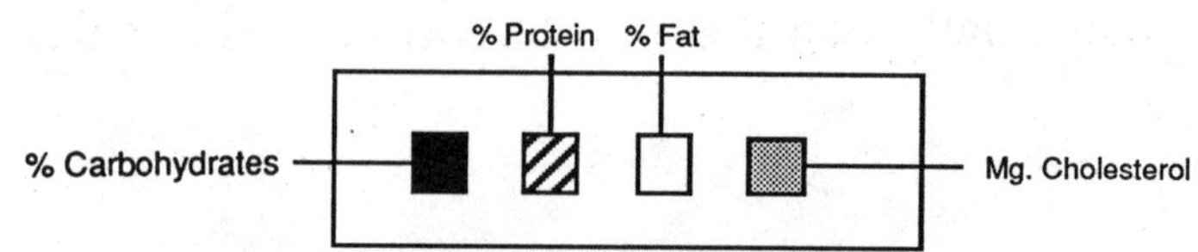

CHOLESTEROL IN 3 1/2 oz. (100 grams) of food (Shown in Mg.)

ORGAN & PROCESSED MEATS

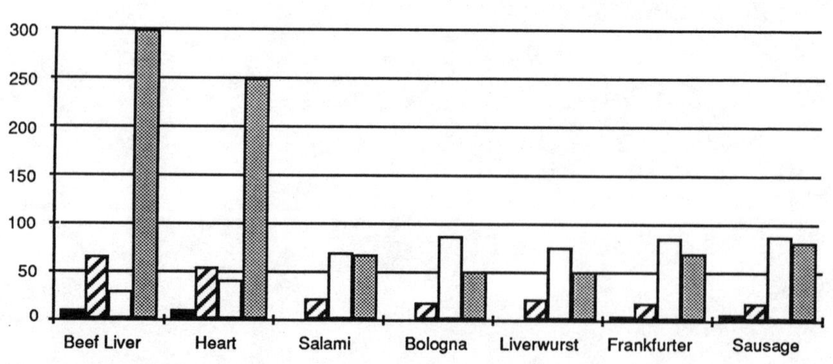

CHAPTER ELEVEN

BREAST CANCER PREVENTION

The principal cause of many cancers is fat in the diet. In studies comparing the amount of fat eaten in different countries, those who eat the most fat - Germany, United States and Denmark - have the highest rate of breast cancer as compared to countries like Thailand, Japan and Spain. Fat intake is closely linked to cancer development, according to Dr. Ernest Wynder, who is the world expert on breast cancer development. Dr. Wynder reported in the December, 1969 issue of "The Cancer Report," "One can plot the incidence of breast cancer against any number of environmental factors. The one correlation that shows up well and may be of etiological significance is between breast cancer and the fat intake of women in various countries of the world."

Excessive dietary fat is the principal cause of breast cancer, which is the number one cause of death in women, age 35 to 55. It takes even more lives than hardening of the arteries or heart disease. This is unfortunate because often breast cancer can be prevented. For example, in Japan those people following a lowfat diet have a very low incidence of breast cancer. Those few who do develop breast cancer are usually found in the inner city where they eat a higher fat diet. When Japanese who follow a lowfat diet migrate to Hawaii, studies show they develop six times the rate of breast cancer as they increase the fat on the Hawaiian diet. We know breast cancer is not hereditary. If it were, the Japanese would have the same rate of cancer in all their genetic race, no matter where they lived.

There are three types of noncancerous lumps commonly found in womens breasts. Fibrocystic disease is defined as "lumpy breasts without cancer" and affects half of all women. Fibrodenomas are round, solid, "marble-like" and freely movable, appearing in the late teens and early twenties. They do not disappear by themselves and may enlarge during pregnancy and lactation. These fibro-adenomas are usually benign. A few studies show avoidance of caffeine for at least six months may remove the discomfort and shrink the fibrocystic lumps. Sources of caffeine include:

	MG. PER STANDARD DOSE
DIET PILLS:	
Dexatrim	200
DIURETICS:	
Aqua-Ban	200
STIMULANTS:	
No Doz and Vivarin	200

<u>COFFEE</u>	
Drip, per 5 oz. cup	137
<u>HEADACHE PILLS:</u>	
Cafergot	100
Migrol	50
<u>COCOA:</u>	
1 oz. dry	70
<u>PAIN PILLS:</u>	
Excedrin	130
Vanquish	66
Anacin	64
Midol	64
Darvon	32
<u>TEA:</u>	
5 oz. cup	20-65
<u>INSTANT COFFEE:</u>	
1 teaspoon	27-60
<u>SOFT DRINKS</u>	
Mountain Dew 12 oz.	54
Coca-Cola 12 oz.	45
Diet Coke 12 oz.	45
Tab 12 oz.	45
Shasta Cola 12 oz.	44
Dr. Pepper 12 oz.	40
Pepsi 12 oz.	38
<u>CHOCOLATE:</u>	
1 oz.	35

DECAFFEINATED COFFEE
OR TEA:

6 oz.	3-5

The second kind of noncancerous lump appears between the ages of 30 to 39. They may fluctuate in size with the menstrual cycle; often they are sore or tender, appearing as an unusually distinct area, and are due to normal variations of breast tissue.

The third type of benign lumps are called cysts, which are firm, fluid-filled sacs and are usually painful. These appear around age 40. 90% of women develop cysts if they have used oral contraceptives longer than two to four years.

CANCEROUS LUMPS

Cancers are hard lumps, usually, not tender and may be either movable or fixed to the skin or underlying tissue. In postmenopausal women, past the age of 45, a newly detected lump such as this should be biopsied. A mammogram is not sufficient to tell if the lump is malignant and cancerous (composed of mutated cells which spread and grow).

BREAST CANCER PREVENTION

The forerunner to cancer is a condition of "hyperplasia" that means "overgrowth." In this situation, cells lining the milk ducts change their appearance, multiply and build up in a cluster inside the duct. In this early stage, a lump is not yet present and the build up of cells does not inevitably lead to cancer. This whole process is reversible up to this point. But, as the condition progresses, the cells may increase in size while becoming more irregular in appearance. Eventually, abnormal cells may plug the duct and then go on to break out of the duct, turning into an invasive cancer.

From autopsy findings, we can predict that of the 30% of women who develop hyperplasia, most them will not get cancer. Yet many women undergo mastectomies (total removal of breast tissue) as if the condition was cancer. This is a tragedy leading to unnecessary psychological suffering and physical disfigurement. This needless surgical approach also distorts the treatment statistics by including women who really didn't have cancer to begin with and mixing them in with true cancer cases. This results in false claims by surgeons of improved life expectancy. Incredibly, some women undergo preventive mastectomies simply because a relative had a history of breast cancer. We have seen no change in the survival rate in 1988, compared to the survival rate as far back as 1950. Surgery, radiation and chemotherapy have almost failed to make any difference.

Early detection with mammogram doesn't solve the problem either, because a breast tumor must be about the size of a pea before it shows on a mammogram. By that time, the tumor has been growing for at least ten years (Guilliano, P., Cancer; 39:2697, 1977). In 90% of the cases, the cancer cells have already entered the bloodstream and started to spread to the other organs of the body. So, early detection, followed by mastectomy, chemotherapy and radiation usually will not cure the woman because cancer of the breast doesn't kill. However, the spread of cancer to the brain, liver or lungs would most likely take the life 10 to 20 years later.

Cancer experts Dr. Ernest Wynder and Denis Burkitt, M.D. have searched for the prevention and eventual cure of breast cancer. A reduction of fat, cholesterol and protein, and an increase in fiber in the diet may be the answer. They believe excess fat in the diet increases the production of certain hormones that may promote the development of breast cancer. Excess fatty acids in the breast tissue increase the production and secretion of the hormone prolaction. Prolactin regulates growth of breast cells and the amount of circulating estrogen. High fat foods like oil, cheese, meat, eggs, cream and milk reach the intestines where bacteria produces even more estrogen. High levels of estrogen increases the growth of breast tissue and the risk of tumors. Breast cancers produce unusually large Amounts of prostaglandins (10 times more than normal breast tissue does). This hormone-like substance also is increased in the body when large amounts of processed essential fatty acids that are found in polyunsaturated vegetable oils such as corn, sunflower or safflower oil are consumed.

Women on a high fat diet menstruate as early as age 12 and begin menopause by age 50. By comparison, women in Thailand and Japan on a traditional low-fat, high starch complex carbohydrate diet start menstruation after age 26, begin menopause at age 46 and have the lowest rate of breast cancer in the world. This was true particularly before 1945. Since WWII, the Japanese diet has become higher in fat. When women from Thailand and Japan migrate to the U.S. and eat a high fat diet, they lose their immunity to breast cancer, developing equally high levels as American women. We know breast cancer is not genetic. It is related to fat in the diet.

Women on a low-fat diet have lower ideal estrogen levels, have lighter and shorter menstrual periods and have less or no pain associated with premenstrual syndrome. Lower estrogen levels reduce the formation of fibroid tumors in the muscular tissue of the uterus. Women with breast cancer have been given Tomoxifen hormone (antiestrogen drug), which has been shown to shrink tumors and improve survival as the estrogen levels are reduced. We also see a lessening of the pain and lumps of fibrocystic breast disease. Contrary to popular belief, we know breast cancer is not caused by a blunt object striking the breast.

We have also discovered malignant cells are unable to manufacture their own cholesterol (normal cells produce as much cholesterol as needed). Yet, when we analyze malignant tumor cells, they have even more cholesterol and fat than normal cells. The cancer cell needs to get its cholesterol from the host, and if you eat foods containing cholesterol, you will provide a generous supply. When we remove cholesterol from the diet to less than 50 mg. a day on the Delgado Health Plan, the cancer tumors may shrink in size and disappear. A cancer cell can take the cholesterol and metabolize it into estrogen. It then uses the estrogen to stimulate growth in the surrounding tissue to spread throughout the body. Women or men can develop breast cancer if given female estrogens, because estrogen stimulates the sex organs and produces abnormal growth.

BREAST CANCER PREVENTION

The fats from oils, cheeses, meats and whole dairy products enter the body and cause an increase of bile acid production in the intestines, which releases an excess amount of estrogen throughout the body. There is also an increase of a hormone called prolactin, which can increase naturally during pregnancy. However, prolactin in excessively high levels has been correlated with the high rate of breast cancer. Women who have breast cancer generally have high prolactin hormone levels. We have discovered, fortunately, women with this high hormone level who reduce fat in their diet can reduce their prolactin and estrogen to safer levels within thirty days. This reduces the risk of breast cancer by 90%, according to Dr. Ernest Wynder. If you are trying to avoid this dread disease, breast cancer, switch to our low-fat, high complex carbohydrate diet.

Not long ago, I came across an article in the L.A. Times that was very upsetting. It reported some women were trying surgery as a preventive measure against breast cancer. I read the subheading and it stated, "Sharon Hughes - I haven't regretted it at all." She was encouraged to have a mastectomy - removal of the breast tissue - because her relatives had breast cancer, and although she showed no signs of the cancer at all, she volunteered to have this surgery done! If the physician in charge had been aware breast cancer is not hereditary, but is related to a high fat diet, she would have had a much better life knowing she could have prevented cancer naturally.

We believe the risk of breast cancer can be reduced by as much as 90% in only 30 days time following a Delgado Health Plan approach - less than 20% calories from fat and more than 70% calories from complex carbohydrates.

The regular daily exercise plan we recommend also may reduce the risk of breast cancer by increasing oxygen levels and reducing the circulating triglyceride fats in the blood.

A high fiber diet also may increase the excretion of estrogen by 2 to 3 times in the feces as compared with low fiber diets of animal products. Women who eat meat have 50% more estrogen in their bloodstream than vegetarian women. Obesity increased the production of estrogen and the risk of breast cancer. The Delgado Health Plan can help you to reach your ideal body weight.

A small, but growing number of women are switching to our low-fat diet approach for treatment to control and possibly reverse cancerous tumors. It is unfortunate research money has only been given to large drug companies for chemotherapy (which has been unsuccessful in women who get breast cancer after menopause), to surgeons comparing which surgery is best and to mammography detection centers.

We strongly advise all women diagnosed with breast cancer to follow a low-fat diet. One out of every ten American women will get breast cancer (120,000 new cases annually and increasing). Major cancer societies now recommend following our type of plan. There have been cases documented of women overcoming cancer, and diet has been the key factor. If your physician is unfamiliar with our type of approach, California now has an informed consent law that requires a physician to explain alternative methods to surgery and we could offer advise on these different methods.

VEGETABLES & LEGUMES

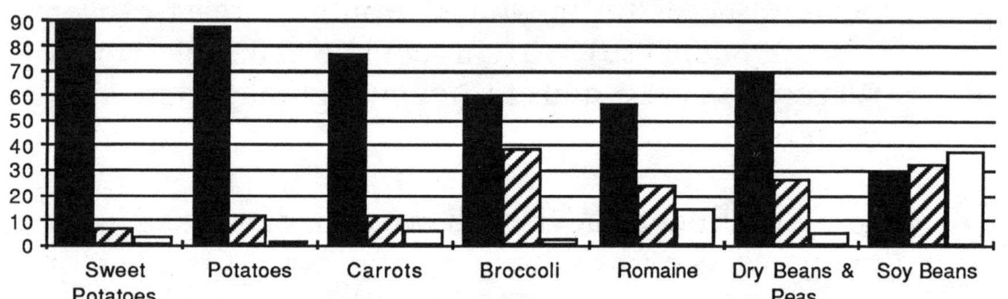

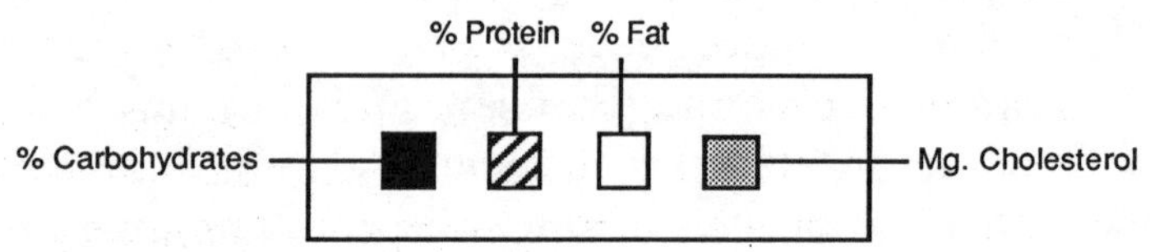

Contains NO Cholesterol

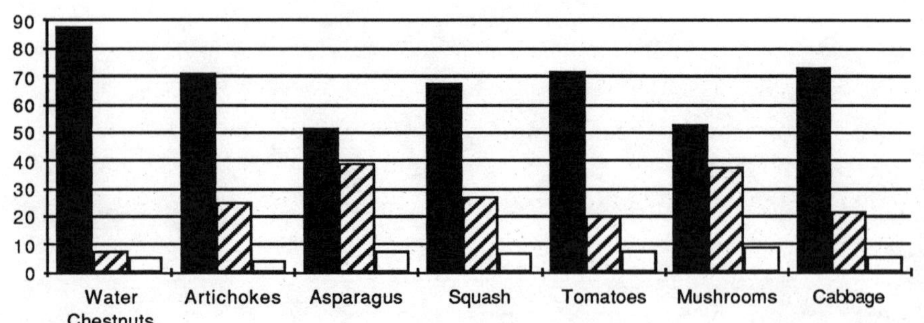

CHAPTER TWELVE

COLON, LUNG, PROSTATE CANCER

The foods we eat in the United States can cause cancer. Colon cancer, for example, is common in the average American. When you eat a high fat diet, there is so much bile acid produced that a bacteria called anaerobic bacteria grows and lives off this bile acid in an oxygen-less environment. Nearly one-third of your total bowel movement is made up of this anaerobic bacteria if you eat the typical American diet. These bacteria give off an excretion called deoxycolic acid, which is a proven carcinogen. This is one of the main reasons the American population is experiencing this increase in the rate of colon cancer.

Many people undergo colostomies to remove the colon, and this is very unfortunate because this type of disease is preventable. When you switch to a low-fat diet, the anaerobic bacteria can no longer live off the excess bile acid. These harmful anaerobic bacteria are pushed out of the body and replaced by good bacteria, called aerobic bacteria, which live in the presence of oxygen. In addition, the high fiber foods are soothing the digestive tract, which increases the intestinal content and actually push out any carcinogenic properties from the body. Remember, if your body passes stools every day, instead of every three days to two weeks, the potential for cancer development is reduced. In countries where they eat the most meat, like New Zealand, United States, Canada and the United Kingdom, they have the highest rate of colon cancer, nearly 40 times higher than in countries like Columbia, Hungary, Nigeria and Japan.

What is being done to prevent and minimize the recurrence of colon cancer in hospitals? An unfortunate example showed us the desperate need for change when President Ronald Reagan had surgery for colon cancer. He was served a hamburger just before his pre-surgery fast, and his first three meals after removal of the cancerous polyp from his colon were: eggs, bacon and buttered toast for breakfast, chicken broth and a cheeseburger for lunch and salmon for dinner - all in the hospital!!

In the early 1950's in Japan, we discovered the rate for colon cancer was very low, less than 3 deaths per 100,000. Yet after World War II, with the dramatic change in their lifestyle, and accompanied by the increase of meat, eggs, fat and milk, there was a significant increase of three to four times the rate of colon cancer. This shows again how colon cancer is related to our lifestyle and the foods we eat.

Of the different types of cancer, lung cancer is the number one cause of death - nearly 70,000 people die every year. Cigarette smoking makes the lungs look black, charred and increases the mutagenic properties.

However, cholesterol is a key factor in the development of lung cancer according to an amazing piece of research by Dr. Jeremiah Stamler. He compared thousands of cigarette smokers, categorized them as moderate or heavy smokers and found those people with the highest cholesterol levels developed lung cancer. This was a shocking discovery.

What did cholesterol have to do with lung cancer? It was always assumed cigarette smoking was the principal cause. In fact, Dr. Stamler showed if a person had a cholesterol level under 150, it made no difference whether the person was a smoker or not. Usually, they did not develop lung cancer. Yet, if their cholesterol was 225-250, or higher, the rate went up to two thousand deaths - a nearly 2000% increase over cholesterol level under 150. If the cholesterol level was over 275, the rate skyrocketed to almost 4,000 deaths. The higher the cholesterol level, the higher the rate of lung cancer.

The correlation between cholesterol and lung cancer has finally been discovered. The lymphocytes (little white blood cells) back up against cancer cells and inject a substance that causes these cancer cells to burst and destroy themselves, while the macrophages (bigger white blood cells) engulf and digest cancer cells. In other words, white blood cells actually can eat viruses and cancer cells. It's been found the body may have developed cancer several times during your lifetime. However, if your white blood cells are active enough, they will protect you and save your life. If you have a high cholesterol level, though, we've discovered the white blood cells become paralyzed (inactive). If a cancer is triggered, for example, by cigarette smoking, asbestos, low oxygen levels in the body or some external factor, the cancer will start to grow. Because the white blood cells are paralyzed, the cancer grows and proliferates until it forms a large tumor and takes your life.

Excess cholesterol causes another problem. Cancerous tumors convert cholesterol into estrogen. As we stated earlier, increased amounts of estrogen in a man or woman's body stimulates the rapid growth of cancer into the surrounding tissue. Cancer cells cannot produce their own cholesterol as normal cells do, they must rely on the host. Studies have shown if you deprive cancer cells of cholesterol, you can shrink the tumor. According the American Journal of Clinical Nutrition (Vol. 37, 1983), the risk of developing lung cancer was directly related to the amount of cholesterol consumed in all five major ethnic groups found in Hawaii. Those people who consumed the least amount of cholesterol rarely developed lung cancer, while those people who consumed the most cholesterol from eggs, meat, organ meats and dairy products had the highest rate of lung cancer.

We know meat is very high in fat content. Also, there is a potential carcinogenic property in beef. Cattle grown on the feed lots grow more rapidly because of the 120 different chemicals given to them. What are these growth hormones, antibiotics and chemicals doing to your body? Isn't it likely some of them are turning into cancer? There are over 20 different chemicals used in our livestock today that have already been identified as carcinogenic. The FDA has banned one of them - DES. Although you may have heard DES causes uterine cancer nearly 20 years after use, they are still discovering quantities of DES in meat eaten by the public. It's suspected the cattle producers are still slipping DES, this growth hormone, into these animals illegally.

Cholesterol crystals are associated with prostate cancer. Over half the men past the age of 50 in the U.S. have enlarged prostate glands, resulting in obstruction of the urethra and the slowing of the urine. A simple infection of the prostate or a high fat diet can increase sex hormones leading to enlargement. A change of diet and antibiotics, if needed, will reduce the swelling to normal. But, if the enlarged prostate is found to have cholesterol crystals within, then this could develop into prostate cancer. A study of 106 cysts (cysts are cocoon encasings of fibroblasts spun by your body around foreign objects that your white blood cells were unable to remove) showed that only 5 were malignant with cancer. The five that were malignant were the only ones with cholesterol crystals.

Experiments have shown when animals were injected with a large amount of cholesterol dissolved in olive oil, it crystalized within the animal and caused malignant cysts to form. When olive oil by itself was injected, some cysts were formed, but no malignancies developed. Plastic cysts were then inserted under animals skin and within two weeks cocoons formed around the foreign object and malignant cells were found inside. If a plastic disc had scratches and holes drilled into it, and then was inserted into an animal, the cocoon formed, but no malignancies could be found. It was discovered the scratches and holes allowed capillaries to take hold and grow inside the cocoon and supply sufficient oxygen to the cells inside, thus preventing cancer. But, the smooth plastic disc and the cholesterol crystals (which are smooth) did not allow enough room for the capillaries to squeeze in as the fibroblasts spun their tight web. This deprivation of oxygen and food causes some cells to die and some to mutate to cancer.

In Canada, three individuals, average age 65 and older, were proven to have prostate cancer. This was verified by needle biopsy. In this procedure, they stick a needle into the prostate and remove cells for testing. The test samples were loaded with cancer. Instead of surgery, these three men volunteered to follow a program that advocated a low cholesterol diet and certain types of cholesterol lowering drug therapy. In essence, they lowered the cholesterol level, and within a period of one month to three years, the cancer had disappeared, confirmed by another needle biopsy. The prostate had shrunk to normal and there was no longer any sign of prostate cancer.

If you think prostate cancer is very easy to cure, you're wrong. It's one of the most serious types of cancers. Years ago, when I worked in physical therapy critical care, I remember a man who had prostate cancer. It was our job to exercise him and keep him as strong as possible. He would exercise up and down the halls and seemed perfectly healthy; the only way we knew he had prostate cancer was from medical tests. He was not provided any special nutritional lowfat diet. He ate the typical high fat hospital food. After only two weeks, he was so fatigued and weak he could barely get out of bed. Two days later he could barely raise his arm. The cancer had grown in the prostate so severely it took away all his energy and it killed him within three weeks.

Dr. Anthony Sattilaro, a physician and president of Philadelphia's Methodist Hospital, contracted a serious case of cancer. According to bone scans, Dr. Sattilaro was diagnosed in May, 1978 with cancerous tumors in his brain, shoulder, ribs and testicles. At first, they did a biopsy, then removed one his ribs and found it was loaded with cancer. They started chemotherapy (drugs) to kill the cancer, and his health decreased rapidly. They removed both his testicles and tried hormone therapy. Since Dr. Sattilaro was a physician in a large hospital, he had access to all the latest therapies and treatments for cancer, but the other doctors gave up and told him he probably would die shortly and he should get his life in order.

According to "Life Magazine" and a follow up book by Dr. Sattilaro, he left his post at the hospital, went for a drive and encountered two young men. He talked with them, told them he had cancer and was going to die. After listening to his story, these young men told the doctor about a special diet that seemed to help those with cancer to live. He didn't believe it at first, after all, he was a doctor and thought he knew everything about cancer therapy. Finally, Dr. Sattilaro decided to follow their suggestion and began following a program that encouraged eating whole grains, vegetables and beans, while avoiding all fats, dairy and animal products.

Because of his changing lifestyle, Dr. Sattilaro started to feel better and the pain throughout his body began to go away. Fourteen months later, a further bone scan revealed all the cancer had disappeared from his body. His body had cleaned itself. How? Dr. Sattilaro reports, with his colleagues, perhaps as his diet was purified, his white blood cells could finally gain enough strength to fight off this serious cancer.

Cancer prevention can be accomplished through a series of steps. You need to reduce your dietary fat intake to under 20%. This is recommended by both the National Cancer Institute and the American Cancer Society. You need to cut cholesterol consumption to under 100 mg. per day. Remember, reduced cholesterol in the bloodstream can improve white blood cell activity, help reduce estrogen production to safe levels and lessen the chance of malignant cocoon formation. Reduce smoked, salt-cured or pickled foods. Switch to lean cuts of meat (chicken, fish or turkey) or, better yet, stop the use of all meats.

Stop cigarette smoking to reduce the exposure to carcinogenic chemicals and the loss of oxygen due to carbon monoxide (see our 7-Day Quit Smoking Program). Next, reduce the use of alcohol. Excessive alcohol intake combined with smoking may be correlated to esophagus cancer (highest in France). Also, chewing tobacco is related to cancers of the mouth. Avoid pollutants, asbestos and additives as much as possible. Reduce the use of peanuts and peanut butter, switching to whole nuts (almonds, cashews, walnuts, etc.) and seeds (sesame, sunflower, etc.) instead.

Eat more fruits and vegetables containing beta-carotene. Beta-carotene foods (which convert into vitamin A as your body needs it) such as carrots, broccoli and brussels sprouts, have a preventive effect on cancer. Those people with high vitamin A levels have a lower rate of cancer than those with a low vitamin A level. Vitamin C rich foods like red bellpeppers, chili peppers, broccoli and strawberries reduce the rate of nitrosamine formation and stomach cancers. Increase the use of whole grains for their fiber content to keep your intestinal tract clean and healthful.

COLON, LUNG, PROSTATE CANCER

The National Cancer Institute is correct in assuming most cases of cancer are preventable. We have seen the benefits of our type of program in the treatment of cancer. Please help us spread the word to your loved ones. Don't depend on current therapies alone; get a second opinion from one of our doctors.

Hospitals are currently using methods considered ineffective for cancer therapy, which all have side effects and may depress your immune system and decrease survival time. For example, a major surgery such as mastectomy should be replaced by a less radical procedure - a lumpectomy, in most cases. This also would reduce the use of blood transfusions. Radiation treatment also may depress your immune system and increase the risk of metastatic disease, according to the medical journal Lancet (2:1285, 1974). Chemotherapy, which is the use of drugs by injection or pills, has been ineffective in prolonging life after cancer develops (Lancet, 2:307, 1984). Lymph node irradiation and lymph node removal is now questioned because lymph nodes produce lymphocytes that help fight cancer, and removal or radiation of the lymph nodes is not beneficial. Finally, the high fat diet served in hospitals worsen the problem.

Don't you think you should start following the Delgado Health Plan? If you have already started our program, stay with it and encourage your friends to contact us for guidance today.

7-DAY QUIT SMOKING PROGRAM

(YOU QUIT ON THE SEVENTH DAY!)

* The desire to quit is most crucial to success.
* You **want** to quit, rather than have to quit.
* 95% of people who have quit smoking employed will power using the steps below on their own!

DAY ONE: Mark off on a calendar 7 days - the seventh day is your quitting day!

DAY TWO: List all the reasons you should want to quit smoking. List all the reasons why you should continue to smoke.

DAY THREE: Record every cigarette you smoke from now until your quitting day. When you notice the urge to smoke, wait a full five (5) minutes before giving in.

DAY FOUR: When you notice the urge to smoke, wait a full ten (10) minutes before giving in. Hold your breath and take deep breaths. (Use any deep breathing exercise you know). Imagine the word STOP or imagine yelling the word STOP.

DAY FIVE: Smoke only when you really want to or must. Cut out all unnecessary times. Purchase only one pack at a time. Never purchase a carton. Use only matches, never a cigarette lighter.

DAY SIX: Cut down to 10 cigarettes today. That is enough nicotine to feel good. Hold nicotine in your system by eating fruit and raw vegetables. Alkaline residue can be maintained by drinking 1/2 teaspoon bicarbonate of soda swirled in a glass of water 2-3 times a day. Calcium carbonate helps too - purchase Tums. Before you go to sleep, repeat your "I QUIT" decision and reasons from step #2 above. Say these in front of a mirror.

DAY SEVEN: THROW OUT ALL CIGARETTES! (Even that last hidden one).
THROW OUT ALL MATCHES! Change routines as necessary.

A. Do not use your smoking chair - rearrange the furniture.
B. Eat lunch someplace else - have a friend join you.

Eliminate the urge to smoke after meals:

* Go for a walk
* Shower
* Avoid coffee, alcohol
* Hold a toothpick in your mouth
* Go to the movies, dance, drive, etc.

There is now a nicotine chewing gum called Nicorette available by prescription. One study found 48% of the Nicorette users were successful in stopping smoking. The gum helps the smoker through nicotine withdrawals by supplying small amounts of the drug without inflicting the lungs with carbon monoxide or any of the 2,000 other chemicals found in tobacco smoke. Once the cigarettes are fully eliminated, it is usually somewhat easy to stop chewing the gum. It's best to cleanse the body of nicotine because it is very addicting. By chewing this gum, the painful "cold turkey" withdrawal effect from nicotine is avoided.

To avoid weight gain, a concern for those trying to stop smoking, eat large amounts of fruits and vegetables and start exercising daily. Finally, develop a positive attitude about yourself and your health. You have only one life. Preserve it - life is precious.

CHAPTER THIRTEEN

ARTHRITIS

Arthritis affects 25% of the United States population. That means 50,000,000 Americans suffer from this painful disease. It accounts for over a billion dollars lost every year through Social Security Disability payments issued to individuals unable to function because of this devastating disease.

One of the most painful forms is gouty arthritis, which generally affects the toe joint first, although it can affect nearly any joint in the body. Gout was very common in the Middle Ages and was at its highest rate in recorded history at that time. Their diet included large amounts of meat - at least six times per day; a typical dish was blackbird pie, a dish in which birds were actually baked in the pie shell!

A sample of blood viewed through a microscope from an individual with gout will reveal sharp crystals. These uric acid crystals attack the joints and cause destruction. It is interesting that these crystals do not destroy the joints directly. Your white blood cells play a role in this destruction.

If your uric acid level is over 7, it is very likely you will develop a gouty arthritis attack. Uric acid is a waste product of nucleic acid found in animal products and high protein foods. A diet high in protein, cheese, other dairy products and animal flesh will cause an elevation of uric acid. If the uric acid level in the bloodstream becomes too high, sharp crystals will form.

Your white blood cells know uric acid crystals should not be in the bloodstream. The white blood cells will begin to engulf these sharp crystals and try to dissolve them. Unfortunately, these crystals are one of the few things in nature the white blood cells cannot overpower. White blood cells can eat and dissolve cancer cells, various bacteria and foreign bodies in your intestinal lining, but they cannot digest uric acid crystals.

Within the white blood cells are little sacks called lysosomes that are the most powerful digestive juices in the human body. When the sharp uric acid crystals puncture the lysosomes, these juices dissolve the outer part of the white blood cell and release into the joint area and begin to dissolve the joint.

Gouty arthritis is one of the easiest problems to cure; you simply reduce the excess proteins in the diet and begin consuming more complex carbohydrates. Within 12 weeks, elevated uric acid levels will lower to a safe range because the crystals begin to dissolve as protein is reduced.

Blood pressure medications will create an artificial elevation of uric acid levels. When Zyloprim or Benamid are prescribed to lower these uric acid levels, other side effects result. It's better to correct the cause naturally and safely by diet.

Rheumatoid arthritis is a more serious form of arthritis. This also involves the white blood cells, but differently than described above. When there is a low oxygen level in the joint area, the white blood cells explode because of a lack of oxygen and release their strong digestive juices, which begin to dissolve the joints.

Medical studies have shown arthritics have a very low oxygen level in the joints. The reason for the low levels is a blockage of red blood cells in the blood vessels that occurs from consuming a high fat diet. A high fat diet is the principal cause of rheumatoid arthritis. The excess fat coats the red blood cells. These red blood cell "clumps" are now too large to squeeze through the capillaries, causing them to become blocked. Imagine how small red blood cells are - a head of a pin can hold five million! Normally, the red blood cells should bounce off each other; but, if there is a large amount of fat in the bloodstream, the red blood cells stick together and form clumps which then create blockages.

When a blockage occurs, the blood fluid keeps pumping and is forced into the surrounding tissues and causes edema. You can literally leave a finger mark or indentation in the skin area affected by edema. Many people with arthritis have edema, but are not aware of it because before edema is visible, one must have a build-up of over 60% fluid.

Edema is also caused by physical trauma. When one is hit on top of the head, a bump forms. This bump is comprised of fluid that accumulates to keep the tissues in place to reduce further destruction. This fluid is so low in oxygen the white blood cells begin to destroy themselves.

One example is "housemaid's knee." A person constantly on their knees will damage the joints. Edema will form because of the accumulation of fluids from trauma and a high fat diet. This fluid accumulation leads to arthritis of the knee because the white blood cells begin to destroy themselves. The same trauma can occur to a construction worker who continually uses a jackhammer to break concrete. The constant vibration leads to arthritis of the fingers.

But, it doesn't always have to be a trauma that leads to edema. We know women have a 200% higher incidence of arthritis than men. As fluids accumulate during the menstrual cycle, the edema concentration, combined with a high fat diet, will cause arthritis.

Another extremely painful type of arthritis is osteoarthritis and is the most difficult to treat. This form of arthritis occurs when the cartilage is damaged due to low oxygen levels. When the white blood cells begin to eat the cartilage, the cartilage seems to alter itself for protection and begins to form itself into bone matter. This will result in bone rubbing directly against bone.

Until recently the only help offered to the arthritis sufferer was anti-inflammatory drugs, including cortisone and aspirin. Although symptoms improve, the deterioration continues within the joints and additional side effects from the drugs may be experienced.

The side effect from aspirin is stomach damage. Cortisone has other side effects after long-term use, including muscle wasting, ulcers, fluid and fat gains. Some pain is reduced temporarily because these drugs suppress white blood cell activity, thus reducing the number of white blood cells left to release their digestive juices. Remember, though, your white blood cells also protect you from disease and infection. With this suppression, you are now susceptible to other problems.

Medical researchers at UCLA extracted white blood cells from the lymph system of patients to treat arthritis. Millions of white blood cells were drained until the symptoms of arthritis were reduced. The patients experienced temporary relief, until the white blood cell count returned to normal and the pain in the joints returned. As you can appreciate, just removing or immobilizing the white blood cells does not address the cause of the problem. We could control this disease if people would recognize arthritis is a result of the high fat foods we eat. For those who believe it is due to heredity, let's examine the Pima Indians.

These Indians live in Arizona, and as a group, consume one of the highest fat diets in our country. Because of this high fat diet, the Pima Indians recorded the highest rate of arthritis in our country, and they also have an extremely high rate of gallstones. (Gallstones are a concentration of cholesterol in the gallbladder, along with an imbalance of polyunsaturated fats. Gallstones can be dissolved by reducing fats and cholesterol in the diet).

We say arthritis is not genetic because the blood relatives of the Pimas, the Tarahumara Indians, consume a high complex carbohydrate diet and have no incidence of arthritis or gallstones. If there were a genetic factor, these people would suffer the same problems.

We have many success stories alleviating the symptoms of arthritis. One of our participants, a ballet teacher, was severely affected. Every morning she had to sit in a hot tub just to move. If she had no help to get to the tub, she would drag herself there. She started the program, avoided fats, increased complex carbohydrates to rid herself of the pain and stiffness. She was fortunate the arthritis had been caught and stopped before the joints had degenerated. There was some scar tissue and some knobby accumulation, but at least further damage was prevented. This woman returned to her teaching and conducted a ballet tour that was extremely important to her career. Later, she went back to school and became a nutritionist by the age of 53.

Another patient, the wife of a chiropractor, was afflicted with a severe case of rheumatoid arthritis though she was only in her early thirties. Her pain and stiffness were eliminated following our recommendations.

I met another woman before I became involved in nutritional research, however, who was not so fortunate. This woman had such a severe case of arthritis that just touching her body would cause tears to roll down her face. Her joints were so crippled her fingers and toes curled under. Her rheumatologist (doctor specializing in the treatment of arthritis) had prescribed several expensive drugs to no avail. Surgery was done on one knee joint and before success could be verifed, surgery was performed on her other knee. Unfortunately, the left knee was left at a 45 degree angle. Her right knee also became totally immobilized after surgery. Her normal breakfast consisted of eggs with bacon and toast with butter. She ate one of the fattiest diets I've ever seen. It was never suggested to her she should change her diet, reduce the large amounts of butter, meat and cheese she was consuming.

The medical dictionaries that are currently available state there is no know cause for arthritis. It is believed by some people arthritis may be caused by some virus. Yet, if the people who prepared the medical dictionaries would do some research and read current literature, they would find the answers are already available. There are enough case studies and world wide studies proving dietary changes can make arthritis a disease of the past.

To reduce the known arthritis forms, it is important to reduce fats in the diet. Begin by consuming more complex carbohydrates. Also, be sure to reduce salt in the diet, because salt causes additional fluid accumulation, which aggravates the arthritis. Exercise will help to reduce fat and fluid accumulation and stress reduction; relaxation techniques also will reduce arthritis symptoms.

If this doesn't give fully immediate relief within seven weeks, investigate allergies to foods. For example, avoid all dairy products, cheese, yogurt and nonfat milk included. In some people milk proteins are not completely digested. Large particles enter the bloodstream where allergic reactions can disrupt the white blood cells and the immune system. Even tiny amounts of milk added to cereal or coffee will cause massive destruction, pain and stiffness in some people.

One lady was cured of arthritis by avoiding all dairy products. However, after only one small serving of a milk product, the pain and stiffness struck her joints within 24 hours! It took her several days of dairy-free eating to recover.

Some people may be allergic to wheat, soybean, eggs, citrus fruit or potatoes. To determine your allergy, eat only brown rice, brown rice cereal or bread, noncitrus cooked fruits, yams and squash. Then gradually introduce one food at a time to test for one week. Eventually you'll discover what foods you must permanently avoid. This is called the "Elimination Diet Method." People have tried rotation diets by rotating foods each week that they are allergic to. This does not work in long term treatment.

Have you heard the suggestion of taking oil to lubricate the joints? Be aware the fluid that lubricates joints is made up of carbohydrates - and oil contains no carbohydrates. The use of vegetable oil or cod liver oil will worsen arthritis!

The best approach to reducing gouty, rheumatoid and osteo-arthritis would be:

1) Improve circulation and reduce edema.
   a) Reduce fats, oils, cheese, fatty meat, etc.
   b) Reduce salt.
   c) Aerobic exercise 4 times per week.

2) Reduce protein (uric acid).

3) Physical therapy, including hot or cold therapy.

4) Restore female hormone balance with exercise and a low-fat diet. (Osteoporosis may be the cause of pain that can worsen if the female hormones are out of balance.)

5) Eat complex carbohydrates, whole grains, beans, fruits and vegetables.

6) Lose weight if necessary.

7) Avoid dairy products for at least 6 months to note any improvements.

8) Identify other allergy producing foods.

If there has already been a degeneration or breakdown of the joints, this cannot be reversed; but, further degeneration can be prevented. Encourage your whole family, young and old, to start following the Delgado Health Plan.

DAIRY FOODS AND EGGS

Avoid Dairy & Eggs since they produce allergies, they're too high in protein, or fat.

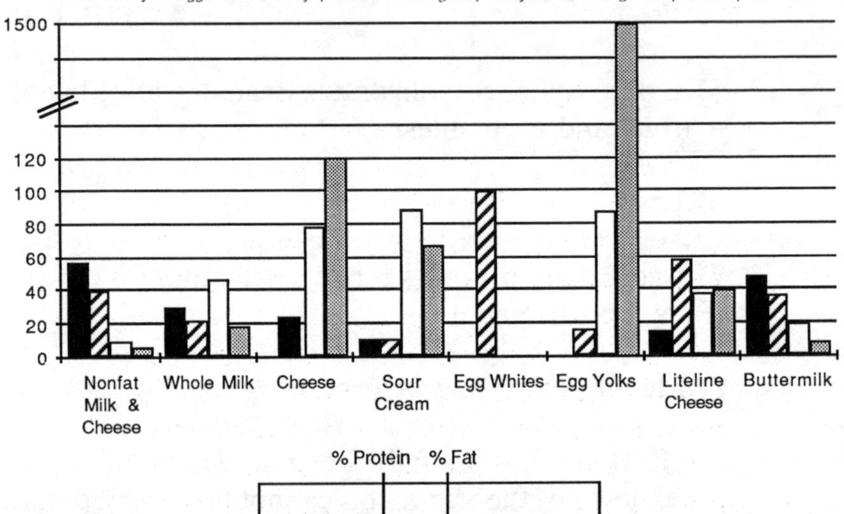

CHOLESTEROL IN 3 1/2 oz. (100 grams) of food (Shown in Mg.)

GRAINS

Eat more whole grains, vegetables, fruit, and beans. They are low in fat and high in fibe

Contains NO Cholesterol

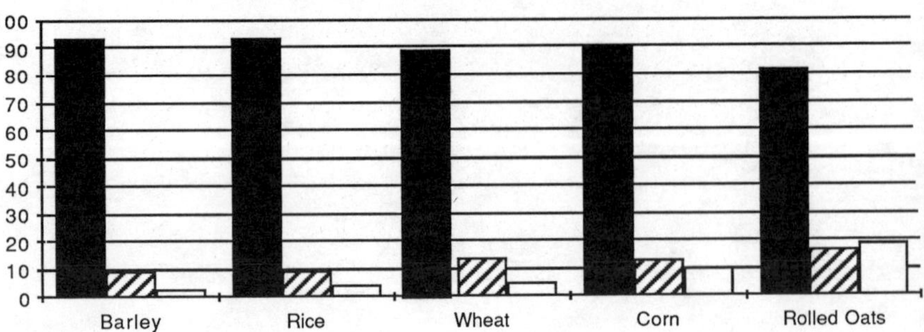

CHAPTER FOURTEEN

DIABETES

There are ten million diabetics in the United States. They are at greater risk of heart attack, stroke, kidney damage, blindness and gangrene, with three times as high a death rate as do nondiabetics. A person is considered diabetic if the blood glucose level after fasting 8 to 12 hours exceeds 130 mg. on two separate occasions. Even after a very large meal, the blood sugar should not exceed 150 mg.

Symptoms of diabetes may include: fatigue, lack of energy, urination at night, constant thirst (you may need water every 15 to 30 minutes to dissolve the overflow of unused sugar in the blood and urine), blurred vision (due to sugar accumulation in the lens of the eye) and weight loss (because of rapid burning of body fat due to your body's inability to use glucose).

Diabetes is mistakenly thought to be "well controlled" by insulin shots or pills. Diabetic drugs can control the blood sugar level, but the drugs have not helped to stop the rapid development of atherosclerosis associated with the diabetic condition. Diabetes is increasing in our country at the rate of 1.5 million new cases developing every year (a 15% yearly increase).

DIABETES

I vividly remember working in the physical therapy department of a hospital where I met a man named Charles. He was intelligent, kind and had a great sense of humor. Unfortunately, he could no longer continue his job as a university administrator because he had become totally disabled by diabetes. He told me he had been at a party and had one drink, and nearly passed out. Everyone thought he was drunk, but later doctors confirmed he had developed diabetes. A year later, he suffered a stroke, and lost the ability to speak clearly (due to brain damage), lost control of his right arm, leg and bowels (he had to wear diapers). Charles became bedridden, and because of the constant pressure on the skin from laying in bed all day, he developed bedsores on his right leg and hip. The nurses tried to keep turning at regular intervals, because anyone who is weak and unable to roll over is in constant danger of bedsores.

Diabetes doesn't allow for proper healing of even minor sores, and before long the doctors had to amputate his left leg - his strong leg - opposite his stroke weakened leg. We were asked to give Charles whirlpool and ultraviolet light treatments for the bedsores on his hip and remaining ulcerated ankle, where you could now see bone and tendons. The doctors struggled to save his remaining leg, but it was no use.

DIABETES

I noticed every morning when I came to help Charles exercise, he was served 2 eggs, white toast with butter and bacon or sausage on the side. His lunches and dinners included large amounts of cheese, meat and dairy products. He was given only small amounts of vegetables and fruits, and even small amounts of whole grains or beans. I tried to tell my patients how important it was to reduce fat in the diet. However, patients in hospitals and convalescent homes are fed a diet based on outdated recommendations. I was unable to have the dietary departments change because I was told state laws had guidelines requiring the "four food groups." This could only be changed with doctors' orders and very few doctors in 1978 were prescribing a low-fat, high fiber diet for patients as treatment.

Now, several years later, we have shown the effectiveness of our program, and more doctors are recommending our approach to their patients. The fact remains, though, millions of people, and especially the ones you love and care about are still unaware of how to achieve this ideal health.

Two scientists, Burson and Yao, won the Nobel Prize after proving a person with diabetes produces as much insulin as a normal person (in 90% of the cases). From this information, we know diabetes is usually not caused by a lack of insulin. We have discovered the principal cause of diabetes is excess fat in the blood, which can desensitize the insulin, and the insulin is then unable to push glucose into the cells for energy. The fat accumulates in the blood from overeating fatty foods such as cheese, butter, margarine, oil, red meat and eggs, and from a lack of regular exercise.

You may develop a temporary case of diabetes for the following reasons:

1) FASTING OVER 48 HOURS - You use your glucose in 12 hours, and then your body is forced to release fat in the blood for reserve energy, just as if you had eaten fat.

2) FEVER - Your body temporarily releases fat in the blood for up to 90 days when you have a fever.

3) STRENUOUS EXERCISE (beyond your capabilities) - This can use your body's storage of glucose, which would trigger the release of fat for replacement energy.

While this fat in the bloodstream can temporarily desensitize the insulin, you don't have to worry about occasionally testing diabetic in these short-lived, mild cases. Serious damage may only occur from years of poor diet or in people who can't produce insulin.

DIABETES

A severe form of the disease called "insulin-dependent diabetes" is caused by the inability of the pancreas to produce insulin in less than 10% of the people with diabetes. The pancreas can be damaged for the following reasons:

1) Excessive long-term use of alcohol - Cirrhotic liver damage from alcohol also can lead to the inability to handle fat, resulting in diabetes.

2) A virus infection, such as the mumps or the flu in some children.

3) Overproduction of hormones by the adrenal, thyroid or pituitary glands.

4) An inherited malfunction of the pancreas.

In these cases, a low-fat diet with exercise can help you to avoid atherosclerosis, blindness and kidney damage that is usually associated with diabetes. You may reduce your need for insulin to body requirements (about 30 units per day), but you probably will need to take insulin for the rest of your life.

You probably will always need insulin if you were started on it before you were thirty years old, if you are very lean and take over 30 units of insulin per day, or if you are very lean and exercise a great deal (for example, run 15 miles/24 km per week or walk briskly 3 miles/5 km per day) and take over 20 units per day. On the other hand, if you are overweight and not very active, with your doctor's help through exercise and weight loss, you can gradually reduce your insulin dose. You may be able to stop your insulin injections with a suitable diet, such as the Delgado Health Plan.

UNDER NO CIRCUMSTANCES SHOULD YOU EVER ATTEMPT TO COME OFF INSULIN EXCEPT UNDER YOUR DOCTORS SUPERVISION.

In a 1935 study of 100 patients, Dr. Rabinowitz, placed half the patients on a low-fat diet (under 20%, as we recommend), and the other half on a high fat diet (56% fat). After the study, it was discovered those on a low-fat diet totally eliminated the need for injected insulin in 24% of the cases and reduced the need for insulin by over 58%. The group on the high fat diet was unable to reduce its insulin at all (less than 1%). The cholesterol levels were also dramatically reduced on the low-fat diet. Dr. Rabinowitz hypothesized it was the low cholesterol, low-fat diet that was the principal reason these diabetics did not develop heart disease, serious gangrene and other side effects, and he was right.

He understood this idea back in 1935! Dr. Rabinowitz tried to convince the American public to change their diet, but no one would believe him. Everyone thought diabetes could not be controlled by diet and you would have to take insulin for the rest of your life.

Another study investigating the cause of diabetes was conducted in 1979 by Dr. James Anderson at the University of Kentucky Medical Center. Dr. Anderson asked his patients to eat one pound of sugar every day for eleven weeks. Can you imagine eating a pound of sugar every day?! That would be like eating one of those five pound containers of sugar in less than a week's time! The rest of the diet was composed of only 5% fat. After the full eleven week testing period, and after checking their blood sugar level weekly, not one person tested diabetic on the glucose tolerance test. The patients' sugar level always measured in the low range; it would have to be over 175 by glucose tolerance to test diabetic. The results were shocking because it was thought sugar caused diabetes.

Afterward, Dr. Anderson tried a diet high in fats (65% fat) with almost no fiber present. In less than two weeks time, every person tested diabetic. He then tried a diet of 45% fat without complex carbohydrates or fiber present and everyone tested diabetic again. He had discovered fat in the diet caused diabetes and not sugar. He then tested a diet with 40% complex carbohydrates and 43% fat. The blood sugar level was higher than the group eating the pound of sugar per day, but it did not get into the diabetic range because the complex carbohydrates with fiber have a protective factor on the insulin itself.

But, if you increase your fat intake for a long period, year after year, one day you'll probably test diabetic. It's assumed people past the age of 65 will eventually become diabetic. This doesn't have to happen. Studies show diabetes does not appear in cultures who follow a low-fat diet throughout their lives.

We strongly recommend you come to our Delgado Clinic to have your blood sugar level checked. If after a fasting test, it's over 100, you're already testing diabetic. If it is 130 or higher, more than likely you're already diabetic. If after eating or having a glucose tolerance test, it goes over 180 and does not return below 100 mg., you are diabetic.

In a second study reported in The Medical Times, May 1980, Dr. Anderson altered the diet of 20 lean diabetics. He selected lean individuals because some doctors would tell their patients to lose weight and the diabetes would be gone. Dr. Anderson discovered weight loss alone wouldn't cure diabetes, although losing weight does help. The diabetics ate a 70% complex carbohydrate, high starch diet for two weeks. Dr. Anderson lowered the fat in the diet and had them eat Shredded Wheat, Grapenuts, crackers, whole wheat, rye bread, beans and raw fruit. The exciting results showed a reduction of insulin by 58% and cholesterol reduction by 30%. Diabetes Outlook also recommended the high complex carbohydrate, low-fat diet to avoid diabetes. The medical journals are coming out with more research showing a whole diet approach is better and safer to use than taking drugs or resorting to insulin.

Past treatments for diabetes have been varied and ineffective; in France they would give people a quarter pound of candy and small amounts of meat. Of course, it didn't help. In England, people were told to eat a high fat diet with no carbohydrates at all. Diabetics were told to eat fat, pork, blood and intestines, as rancid as they could bear. Unfortunately, this increased the death rate of the diabetics. Since they avoided carbohydrates, the doctors thought they were helping the problem!

There has been so much confusion in our country, too, about avoiding carbohydrates as treatment for diabetes. Yet, the Egyptians, 3,500 years ago, knew a low-fat, high complex carbohydrate diet was the best treatment for diabetics. It's written in their hieroglyphics: breads, berries and fruit. The Romans also knew this high fiber, lowfat diet would control diabetes. Dr. Kelly West, world-renowned endocrinologist, has reported over 62% of the adult-onset diabetics could be off insulin and back to normal on this low-fat, high complex carbohydrate diet. Similar results were also reported by Dr. Kempner at Duke University.

The benefits of the complex carbohydrates include increased endurance, greater energy, lowering of blood fats, reduced cholesterol and triglycerides, increased fiber or bulk to the stools and control of the blood sugar level. We know exercise also reduces the blood glucose level by reducing fat in the blood and improves the sensitivity of insulin, whereas bed rest and inactivity causes high blood sugar levels. We also know hypo-glycemia, which used to be treated by a high protein diet, is best controlled by the high complex carbohydrates. The Delgado Health Plan can give you enough blood sugar to control and maintain a high, even source of energy. Eat more potatoes, fresh fruits and vegetables and you'll be rid of hypoglycemia.

In summary, to avoid diabetes we recommend you eat more complex carbohydrates (grains, starches, beans, vegetables and fruit) and reduce the foods that cause diabetes - fats, oils, cheeses and meats. You also should increase aerobic exercise (30 minutes daily is sufficient), visit the doctor regularly if you are on insulin to change the dosages as needed and reduce sugar intake to avoid hypoglycemia (although sugar is not the cause of diabetes, it may lead to hypoglycemia). The major agencies - the Diabetic Association and the Cancer Institute now agree with the Delgado Health Plan to reduce fat to under 20%, increase complex carbohydrates to over 70% and reduce cholesterol intake. We have discovered how to avoid serious degenerative diseases such as diabetes - follow our Delgado Health Plan.

FRUIT

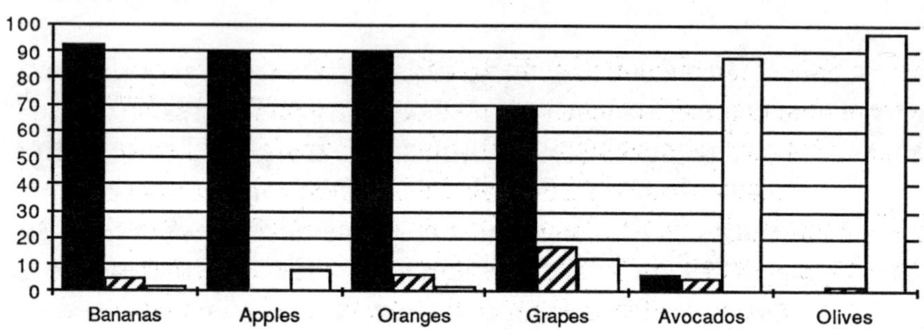

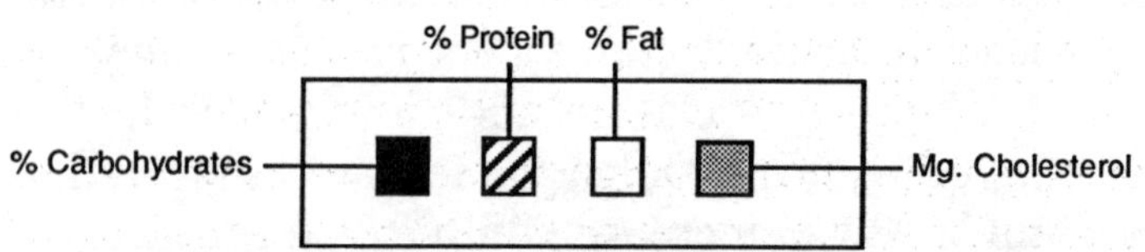

Fruits, vegetables, grains, beans, and sprouted seeds are low in fat, cholesterol, and high in fiber. This must make up the main diet for diabetics and health minded people. Limit the use of avocados, olives, nuts, seeds, and coconut. Avoid the use of any oils, fats, meats, and chee

Contains NO Cholesterol

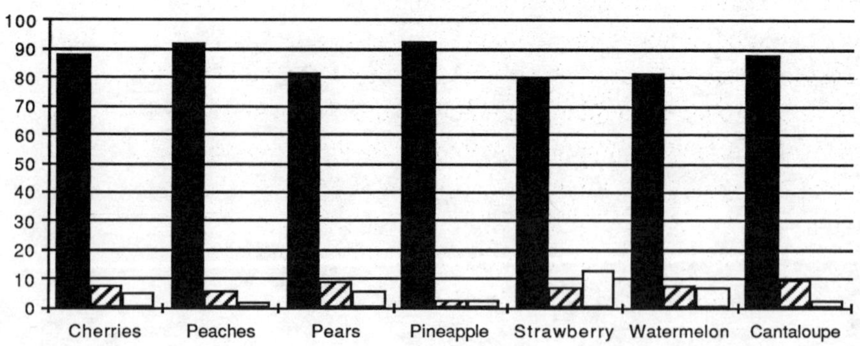

CHAPTER FIFTEEN

DIGESTION

I would like to take you back in time about four million years to understand how to achieve ideal health. Dr. Bryant Van of Texas A&M University studied prehistoric man's diet. The only way to do this was to analyze fecal material. He found primitive man ate primarilary whole grains, vegetables, smaller amounts of fruits, nuts and seeds. Meat was rarely eaten, and only when they could catch some prey. We find the same basic diet over hundreds of thousands of years. Ten thousand years ago, man was still subsisting on grains, fruits and vegetables.

It wasn't until approximately two hundred years ago that large quantities of meat and dairy products entered our diet. There has been a reduction in the use of whole grains, fruits and vegetables since then and a continual increase in cholesterol intake. Within the last thirty years, unfortunately, there has also been an alarming increase in our diet of sugar, salt, fats, food additives and artificial foods. What are we going to see in the coming decades? What will be the health of our future generations? We need to understand the digestive system to grasp these problems.

DIGESTION

The digestive process begins when you chew food and the salivary glands secrete saliva to help break down the food. It then goes down the gullet to the stomach where it encounters certain digestive enzymes. Next, it passes through the small intestine and is broken down further by digestive juices secreted by the pancreas, gallbladder and liver. The food goes down a long pathway in the small intestine, nearly 32 feet, where there is a tremendous absorption area. The little villi located here absorb much of the food, with the remainder moving to the large intestine and eventually passing out of the body.

When we talk about the food we eat, an analysis of packaged food labels of 10 years ago would show the term "crude fiber" was often used. This was an inaccurate measurement of the actual fiber content in food because they would boil the food in the presence of a weak acid or alkali. All that remained was cellulose and lignin and it was believed this was the amount of fiber in food. This was a critical mistake, though, because "dietary fiber," the term we now use, is truly the total amount of plant food remaining intact and undigested after passing through the small intestine. What we find remaining is not only cellulose and lignin, but also pentose, pectin, guar gums, bengal gram, etc. There are several different components to fiber itself.

Fiber acts like a sponge, retaining water as it passes through the small intestine. This is usually called roughage, which is a misnomer because it gives the impression the food you eat roughs up the intestinal tract. Instead, we should call it "softage," because as this undigested food passes through the lower digestive system, it acts like a sponge to absorb water and other fluids, creating large, soft stools that pass out of the body in a healthy manner.

If we ingest a radioactive isotope (enclosed in a tiny case), we can monitor its intestinal transient time (the amount of time it takes to pass through and out of the body). Generally, in a healthy individual it should pass out within 1 1/2 days. The shocking truth is for the average American, the transient time is over three days, and as long as two weeks in many elderly people! We then have the resultant health problems.

One problem which develops is the result of a large amount of intestinal pressure inside the abdomen, created as fiberless food passes through the digestive tract and pulls out all the fluid. As a result, you're left with little, hard, rock-like stools, which some people call "bullets" or "buttons". This problem is wide-spread because of the preponderance of animal products (meat, cheese, eggs, dairy products, etc.) in our diet. These foods are all totally digestible, and devoid of fiber. You need about two hundred grams (7 ounces) of intestinal content to reach the rectum and pass out of the body. If there is less than this amount, (the average American has only about 3 ounces) the body has to use all its pressure and muscles in the abdominal area to force these stools out of the body.

As a result, one of the problems which will develop early on is hiatus hernia, a condition in which the upper part of the stomach is pushed up through the diaphragm toward the thoracic area. This is the most common cause of heartburn because the gastric juices pool in this area and burn. We now know the hiatus hernia is clearly related to constipation. We also know hiatus hernia is not present in cultures which follow a high fiber diet.

Gallstones can also develop from lack of fiber in the diet. The gallbladder, which contains bile salts and cholesterol, sprays these bile salts and substances over the food to help digestion. If there is a lack of dietary fiber, large concentrations of cholesterol develop in the gallbladder. Of course, we also develop high concentrations of cholesterol from eating high cholesterol foods and gallstones, usually, are made of cholesterol in crystalized form.

These stones can be dangerous because severe pain can result if they block off the little passageway from the gallbladder to the intestines. It's probably one of the most severe pains a person could ever experience, and is sometimes mistaken for appendicitis. The removal of the gallbladder is the most common operation in the U.S., approaching 500,000 yearly. The gallbladder is simply a collecting sack for bile from the liver. Removing the gallbladder does not solve the problem because stones can still form and lodge in the passageway between the liver to the intestines. This could lead to jaundice and some very serious side effects.

We have found if you increase fiber in the diet, while also decreasing cholesterol and fat intake, the following will happen:

1. The fiber, especially water-soluble fiber, removes cholesterol from the body and the intestines. This helps to keep the balance of cholesterol to bile salts equal.

2. Fiber pulls more bile salts out of the body, which means instead of returning to the liver, the liver cholesterol has to be converted into additional bile salts.

3. A large intake of wheat fiber or water-insoluble fibers found in all types of grains, increases the production rate of a solvent, called cheno-deoxycholate, which helps to keep these gallstones dissolved.

Most people do not realize that gallstones can be dissolved instead of resorting to surgery. We have found diet can dissolve these gallstones, especially if they're caught in the early stages. We know of several patient case reports where gallstones have successfully dissolved. If you have stones, have your doctor monitor your progress with the appropriate ultrasound or X-ray tests. Give yourself time and follow the Delgado Health Plan very closely.

Another common digestive disorder is appendicitis. The appendix, located near the end of the large intestine, looks like a little finger. We find the appendix often becomes infected in young people. It's the most common emergency surgery done in this country. It occurs more commonly in young people because the appendix is much more narrow at a younger age. As you get older, it enlarges somewhat. If a young person suffers from a viral infection, the lymph also swells up because there is more lymph tissue in the appendix. If you are eating a low-fiber diet, without natural whole foods, the fecal material becomes so hard it can be trapped in the appendix and possibly lead to a serious infection, which is the cause of most appendicitis cases.

When I was in my early 20's, I was rushed to the hospital with incredible pain. All I could think was, "Whatever you have to do to get rid of this pain, do it!" They removed my appendix, which was severely infected, and later told me they had saved my life on the operating table. I wish I had known ahead of time I could have prevented this painful experience through a whole, natural diet. I don't think any of you would want to go through this surgery, either. We suggest, therefore, young people start the program right away. Appendicitis can be prevented by following a high fiber, "softage" diet. Food will not be trapped in the appendix, and because there is no hard fecal material, there is no cause for infection. In Third World countries, appendicitis rarely, if ever occurs because of their diet.

Another digestive disorder, also resulting from a lack of fiber, is diverticulosis. This disease affects one out of every three adults past the age of sixty, and one out of ten younger people. It occurs when the intestinal tract begins to form bursts or bubbles along the way. Constipation leads to high pressure inside the intestine that forms bubbles along the walls called diverticuli. Although this does't always lead to serious side effects, sometimes it can become infected and then you have a problem called diverticulitis. But, this also can be avoided by increasing natural fibers in the diet.

Research studies now show when you increase the fiber, it reduces the pressure in the intestines, and often there is no need for surgery. This is an exciting development - to know we can avoid the serious consequences related to diverticulosis. Unfortunately, some doctors still recommend a low-fiber, bland diet for diverticulosis and this is a very dangerous mistake.

Over 50% of the American population suffers from hemorrhoids, or piles. We always hear jokes about hemmorrhoids and commercials for hemorrhoid relief, but it's serious if you have them. The process leading to this condition begins at the soft, anal cushion near the end of the rectum that is there to retain the fecal material at appropriate times. But, if you build up pressure in the intestines from lack of fiber, the constant pressure leads to a swelling of the blood vessels in this anal cushion. When hard, fecal material (which should be soft) passes by, the shearing pressure pushes these enlarged blood vessels and anal cushion out to the external part of the body. This can lead to itching, infection and very serious cases requiring surgery.

Fortunately, here again, we have found the increase in fiber in the diet can relieve this extra pressure, and sometimes avoid the need for surgery. "Preparation H" and other similar products do not get to the cause of the problem as does dietary fiber. Ulcerative colitis and spastic colon are also caused by a lack of fiber and worsened by allergies to dairy products or other foods. Try a high fiber diet centered around the least allergy producing foods like whole grain brown rice, yams, squash and cooked noncitrus fruits. Then, each week add back in other grains, vegetables and fruits to identify foods that cause you digestive upset.

Varicose veins are another problem caused by a low-fiber diet. Over 50% of men and women past the age of fifty have these unsightly veins throughout their legs. Usually they occur in the blood vessels in the leg are located very near the skin, and are not surrounded by muscle to help maintain support. When pressure is built up in the intestines from constipation and straining to evacuate hard fecal material, the blood in the veins gets pushed back. This pressure damages the valves that are designed to allow blood to flow up toward the heart again; if these one-way valves get pushed backward, all the blood pools in the veins, causing them to distend and become swollen and very unsightly.

The high fiber, natural foods help to prevent the formation of varicose veins. But, once they do form, it questionable whether they can be reduced because of the severe valve damage in the vein. In that case surgery is usually done or they tie off the flow of that vein. Varicose veins are preventable, and if they have already developed, the Delgado Health Plan can prevent further occurrence and development of these unsightly veins.

It should be noted varicose veins are not present in other cultures. Many people believe varicose veins are caused by pregnancy, but in cultures where the women give birth to as many as nine children, such as the Bantus of Africa, varicose veins don't occur. The Bantus eat a high fiber, natural diet that prevents this pressure build-up. Some people have suggested standing on your feet all day causes varicose veins. Barbers, who stand all day, were compared to other groups who don't stand regularly, and no greater incidence of varicose veins was found. Of course, standing may irritate the situation somewhat, but a high fiber diet makes a difference in our digestive tract.

If you are having problems passing a large, soft stool at least once or more each day, or if they are hard, rock-like stools, begin adding at least one heaping tablespoon of wheat bran to your daily diet.

Sprinkle it in your whole grain cereal or soup, and within one week you should see improvement. If there is no improvement, then add another tablespoon after the first week; by the end of the third week you may have to add another. Keep adding fiber until you find how much is needed to maintain regularity.

Many people believe they eat a high fiber diet because they eat salads. Salads are very high in water content and low in fiber. The best source of fiber is wheat bran, which is very concentrated. Buy the coarse type of Miller's wheat bran which does the job much better than the fine type of bran. The second best sources would be the whole grains: brown rice, millet, corn, rye, etc. Next would be the legumes group, including beans, peas, nuts and seeds. Root vegetables such as carrots, potatoes and parsnips are the fourth best sources of fiber. The fifth, and least sources of dietary fiber would be fruits and vegetables.

Americans have increased their dietary intake of fruits and vegetables, thinking they are now getting enough fiber. In reality, those are the poorest sources of whole fiber. Highly processed foods with no fiber - dairy products, meats, cheeses, oils and animal products are harmful to your health. Eat a high fiber, natural diet for good health.

MEAL PLAN

You may substitute any fruit, vegetable, grain of your choice. To lose fat weight- eat more vegies & fruit.

MEAL	SUNDAY	MONDAY	TUESDAY	WEDNESDAY	THURSDAY	FRIDAY	SATURDAY	INSTRUCTOR'S COMMENTS
BREAKFAST Drink 2-4 glasses of water just before →	Oatbran cereal with apple juice and raisins. Whole wheat toast with apple butter. Exercise	Old fashioned oatmeal with cinnamon. Four prunes. Exercise	Cracked wheat hot cereal with berries ½ grapefruit Exercise	Nutrigrain cereal with soy milk and sliced banana. Oat bran muffin Exercise	Wheatena hot cereal with chopped apple and cinnamon. Exercise	Perkey's nutty brown rice cereal. 1/2 grapefruit Chamomile tea Water Exercise	Pancakes (multi-grain) with blueberry syrup (no sugar) and dry (without oil) hashbrowns. Exercise	All breads, cereals, pastas are wholegrain. All cereals without sugar or honey (use fruit). Any dairy products are nonfat. All water between meals.
10:30 SNACK	Water, Banana	Water Grapes	Water Granny Smith apple	Water Nectarine	Water Red Delicious apple	Water Orange	Water Orange	All tea is herbal. All fruit is whole and fresh.
LUNCH	Whole wheat pita bread with lettuce, sprouts, tomatoes, raw vegetable sticks. Water	Split pea soup over baked potato, veggie sandwich on 7 grain bread. Carrot sticks. Peach Smoothie	Eggplant sandwich with wholegrain bread, lettuce and alfalfa sprouts. Jicama sticks Banana Sundance cranberry sparkler.	Whole wheat pita bread with brown rice, corn, peas, lettuce and chopped fresh parsley. Raw zucchini and carrot sticks. Water	Burrito - Whole wheat or corn tortilla with artichoke hearts (water-packed) Precooked potatoes, beans; microwaved with salsa and sprouts.	Sliced, ripe banana sandwich on whole wheat bread with applebutter. Raw broccoli and caulifloweretes. Water	Mexican salad; lettuce, kidney beans, tomatoes, in wholegrain pita bread; with alfalfa sprouts. Sundance apple sparkler.	All preparations are without oil, fats, margarine. "Hold the mayonnaise." Use Hains natural mustard. Water is between meals.
3:30 SNACK	Mineral water Tangerine	Golden Delicious apple	Bran muffin with unsweetened applebutter	Sundance orange sparkler Melon	Fresh pineapple chunks	Mineral water Pear	Peach	All salads are with no oil dressing or lemon juice.
DINNER	Baked potato with chopped broccoli. Baked bellpepper stuffed with brown rice, mushrooms, onions. 3 Bean Salad	Baked, sliced eggplant in meatless spaghetti sauce over baked zucchini, veggi-pasta casserole. Brown rice with corn and green peas.	Wholegrain elbow macaroni with sliced zucchini and carrots in butter buds. Steamed green beans. Chopped broccoli	Wholewheat spaghetti with mushroom spaghetti sauce. Steamed cauliflower Baked potato with lemon juice and chopped parsley	Baked spaghetti squash with spaghetti sauce. Corn on the cob Lentil soup with chopped fresh parsley on top. Steamed asparagus	Enchiladas stuffed with brown rice, pinto beans, lifetime cheese, fruit ambrosia.	Chinese hot and sour soup, vegetable chow mein, szechuan spicy noodles. Baked Bananas Flambe. Chinese herb tea.	All cooking is without salt and oil. Use herbs for seasoning and water for oil. All water is purified.
APPETIZER AND FRUIT	Raspberry Nouvelle Sorbet	Sundance apple sparkler	Tangerine	Hot air popcorn Red Delicious	Nouvelle Sorbet, strawberries	Hot air popcorn	Strawberry Nouvelle Sorbet	All popcorn is "natural"

CHAPTER SIXTEEN

CHILIES AND SPICES FOR HEALTH

From Cajun cafes to Szechuan Chinese restaurants we are rediscovering the fiery chili peppers. Chili peppers, a surprisingly potent source of certain vitamins, can lower the risk of heart trouble, improve pulmonary function and stimulate the appetite. By loosening congestion, they also may help your next cold. And, they probably don't irritate ulcers, as once thought.

They're a fair source of iron and contain a little magnesium, thiamin, riboflavin and niacin. They are packed with vitamins A and C - the hotter and redder, the better.

Chili peppers can be served as a spice, a condiment or a vegetable. Serve the milder ones as a vegetable and you have a perfect high impact diet food with lots of taste and nutrients for only 24 calories per cup.

Studies in Thailand where hot chilies are eaten at nearly every meal, have shown a reduction in the incidents of life threatening blood clots.

Contrary to popular belief, chili peppers don't seem to hurt ulcers. "There is no data to show that peppers do any harm to the stomach," explains Dr.

Arnold Levy, vice president for education at the American Digestive Disease Society. The stomach protects itself by secreting mucous that coats the lining and shields it from irritants like chilies.

In a British Medical Journal Study, 50 people with ulcers were divided into two groups, Group 1 ate a normal diet without chilies, plus a prescribed antacid. The 25 participants in Group 2 had the same antacid treatment, but consumed red chili powder with every meal. After four weeks, 80% (20 people in each group) had healed duodenal ulcers. Red chilies, they concluded did no harm.

Hot peppers may even improve digestion and stimulate appetite. They increase the production of saliva and gastric juices. That not only helps us digest foods, but sends a message to the brain that food is coming.

Capsaicin, the active ingredient, can be found in a multitude of prepared products - pickled jalapenos, hot sauce, paprika, chili spices. But, nothing compares to the subtle tastes and low sodium content of fresh chilies.

If you take a bite and feel smoke pouring out of your ears, the solution is simple - eat something bland. Bread, potatoes or avocados will help. Water usually makes things worse.

Grow your chilies or buy them fresh. Then dry, can or freeze them for future use. Fresh peppers should be firm with unblemished skins. If wrapped in a paper towel and put in a paper bag, they will last up to four weeks in the refrigerator. If you boil or roast them first, you can freeze them.

Chilies help us enjoy the Delgado low-fat, low sodium, high carbohydrate plan. Make it hot or make it mild and add a little spice to your life.

Chilies: 3 1/2 ounces contain:

Vitamin A 5,000 to 10,000 IU;
Vitamin C 190 - 240 mg.
Sodium 7 mg.
25 - 40 calories

Note: the hotter and redder the chili, the more Vitamin A and C.

Very hot chilies include green hot chili peppers: Serrano (Chili Verde), Habanero, Jalapeno; red hot chili peppers.

Mildly hot: Anaheim (Chili Colorado), Poblano.

Mild, sweet: Red or green bell peppers.

SPICES: From drying and grinding up fresh chili peppers.

Very hot: Cayenne (red); Chipotle (brick red, dried Jalapeno).

Mildly hot: Ancho (ground Poblano pepper in most commercial chili powders); Paprika (ground chili peppers); black, white and pink pepper.

CHAPTER SEVENTEEN

VITAMINS AND MINERALS

Food is the best source to meet your nutritional needs for vitmains and minerals. Only 42 vitamins and minerals have been discovered at this time, and the possibility remains several more will be found. Your best chance of obtaining the nutrition you need would be from whole natural foods like vegetables, fruits, grains, beans and sprouted seeds. Choose a variety of whole natural foods and eat them in quantities sufficient to meet your calorie needs.

Start sprouting seeds, beans, peas, wheat, sunflower seeds, alfalfa seeds, lentils and chick peas. Sprouting helps reduce the fat content of the seeds. It also enhances the protein and enzyme quality of the food so it is fresh and alive. Live food may include certain necessary nutrients we have yet to understand fully.

Sprouting is simple - place a teaspoon up to a quarter cup of seeds into a glass jar. It's best to use glass instead of plastic because the light coming through the glass affects the growth beneficially. A wire screen or a cheesecloth cover works well. Add water and let the seeds soak overnight. Pour off the water the next day. Then, rinse the seeds with fresh water once or twice a day, perhaps in the morning and again at night. Leave the jar at a 45 degree angle after you pour out the water. Keep it in a dark area or in indirect light, since the sprouts grow best in this situation. Sprouts are ready to eat by the fourth day. Usually you can start a new jar one day, start another one the next and so on, for a constant supply of fresh sprouts. They're great for stuffing in sandwiches and salads. Sprouting can increase vitamin and mineral content of the food from fifty to nearly two thousand percent, especially for many B complex vitamins and vitamin C.

Many nutritionists are trained by professors advocating the outdated four food groups and by textbooks (prepared from studies paid for by the meat and dairy industry). The use of liver, eggs, cheese and meat are not good sources of vitamins and minerals because of the excess fat, protein and cholesterol content. Do not be misled into believing you need these harmful foods for "proper nutrition".

You may need to use supplements with our program, but only if you're eating processed foods, white flour, sugar or alcohol, or if you live in a polluted environment. Who doesn't have these situations? They are very common. In other words, we know you're going to cheat on occasion. You might want to take a vitamin-mineral supplement as a preventive formula. You want a multiple vitamin and mineral that at least meets the RDAs (possibly with more B complex, if you drink alcohol or get more sugar in your diet than you want). You need to understand safe ranges because too many supplements can be toxic. The following is a guideline of vitamins and minerals found in foods and their role in good nutrition.

VITAMIN A

This substance comes from either animal or vegetable sources. The animal source of Vitamin A is somewhat toxic, especially if you take in 100,000 international units (I.U.) per day. In a four month period, it was shown to cause nerve, bone and cartilage damage. It has been known to halt growth in children, lead to blurred vision, headaches, hair loss and to force cholesterol deposits into the tissues. A deficiency of Vitamin A, however, has led to an eyeball disease, blindness of the eye and aged skin. We can avoid both problems, getting too much or too little, simply by relying on the vegetable source of Vitamin A, betacarotene, because you cannot overdose on the vegetable source.

For example, a cup of carrots has about 16,000 I.U. of Vitamin A, and a cup of sweet potatoes about 20,000 I.U. The Recommended Daily Allowance (RDA) is only about 5,000 I.U. Somewhere between 5,000 and 15,000 would meet anyone's needs. If you ate too many carrots, sweet potatoes, mustard greens or squash, eventually your skin may turn a little orange or yellow. Once your body is ready to convert the betacarotene underneath the skin into Vitamin A, it will; there is no toxicity known with vegetables, so it is perfectly safe to eat them in large quantities. We want you to avoid the animal sources of Vitamin A as much as possible. Liver, egg yolks and butter fat are high sources of Vitamin A and can be toxic. This source of Vitamin A can build-up in your tissues and lead to side effects and of course, these foods also contain cholesterol. Most yellow and orange-colored vegetables and fruit, such as cantaloupe, contain the safe type of Vitamin A (beta-carotene). Our Delgado Health Plan supplies more than enough Vitamin A, and certainly more than the typical American diet.

RDA: 5,000 I.U.

Animal source supplement not to exceed 10,000 I.U. Vegetable source (beta-carotene) is your best choice; toxicity has only been reported from the animal sources.

1 CUP	I.U.
Hot, red chili peppers	23,500
Sweet potatoes, mashed	20,150
Carrots, cooked	16,280
Pumpkin	16,000
Collards	14,820
Mustard spinach	14,760
Butternut squash	13,120
Dandelion greens	13,000
Carrots, raw	12,100
Seaweed, nori	11,000
Garden cress	10,400
Kale	9,000
Turnip greens	8,000
Winter squash	8,000
Mango (1/2)	7,920
Swiss chard	7,830
Beet greens	7,400
Amaranth, grain	6,100
Muskmelons	5,440
Parsley	5,100
Red bell peppers	4,450
Cantaloupe	4,304
Broccoli	3,880
Apricots (3 average)	2,890

VITAMIN E

Vitamin E is important to prevent rancidity. It helps the oxygen in the body and protects the cells. Vitamin E is also necessary on a low-fat diet, however, people following a high fat diet tend to require more. If you take Vitamin E as a supplement, it's best not to exceed 400 I.U. It was found at 600 I.U., there is an increased rate of triglycerides (fat) in the blood because Vitamin E is a fat. If you break open a capsule, you'll see fat. The dry form of Vitamin E turns into fat, also. Fifteen micrograms, which is much more than the RDA, has been known to lead to weakness and fatigue.

At this time some claims made about Vitamin E are not clear and are not accurate. It is true we need Vitamin E, but it would be better to get it from whole natural foods. For example, kale, cucumbers, or collards contain Vitamin E. Cucumbers contain about 8 I.U. per cup; two cups would complete your entire requirement for the day. Summer squash, millet, green peas and various other fruits and vegetables provide sufficient Vitamin E.

RDA: 15 I.U.

Best not to exceed 400 I.U./day. If you reduce fat in your diet, Vitamin E is used more efficiently.

1 CUP	I.U.
Collards	15.00
Cucumbers	8.40
Kale	8.00
Summer squash	7.50
Millet	4.00
Turnip greens	3.40
Whole wheat flour	3.12
Green peas	3.00
Asparagus	2.60
Herring	2.30
Hazelnuts (6)	1.80
Mango (1/2)	1.50
Almonds (6)	1.33
Whole wheat bread (3)	1.00
Banana	1.00
Leeks	1.00
Chestnuts	.80
Mushrooms	.60
Celery	.57
Tomato	.54
Onions	.44
Grapefruit	.26

VITAMIN B-12

B-12 is part of the B complex family and is necessary to good health. The B complex vitamins help your body to use carbohydrates, to burn them for energy and to use the protein and the fat you eat. Vitamins should not be taken without food because they are like an enzyme that helps to put the food to use. Some people fast or skip meals and then take vitamins believing they're helping themselves. If you do take vitamin supplements, you should take them with your food, or else you should depend on your food as your nutrient source.

Vitamin B-12 deficiencies could result in pernicious anemia. Only a few cases of dietary B-12 have been reported in scientific literature, and those cases were associated with intestinal disorders. If there was an absorption problem, there would be an intrinsic factor enzyme that would be absent because of a disease of the stomach or small intestines. In that event, although you were getting enough B-12, you may not be able to absorb it and you may need an injection once every three months. Equally effective, according to the British Medical Journal (291:56,1985), would be one large daily dose, 1000 mcg., in a pill. A diseased body could absorb the needed 1-2 mg. per day, which would solve the problem. Doctors can diagnose possible Vitamin B-12 deficiencies with blood tests through reports on the complete blood cell counts (CBC) and the anemia panel, which measures the level of Vitamin B-12, folic acid and iron. The live blood morphology test can identify B-12 deficiencies. The red blood cells become shaped like an oval (ovalocytes) instead of being round. Excess B-12 has not been reported as a toxic problem. Many vegetarians take Vitamin B-12 in a B-complex twice or three times a week.

You do need at least four micrograms per day, which is a very small amount. Since your body can store Vitamin B-12 from five to ten years in the liver, we have an adequate storage capacity. B-12 is manufactured by certain bacterial algae (no animal or plant produces B-12). Some foods that provide Vitamin B-12 from bacteria would include one ounce of oysters that has five micrograms (your entire B-12 requirement for the day) and two ounces of crab (5.7 micrograms). An occasional bit of oyster or crab sprinkled into your food would give you all the B-12 you need. Two ounces of herring per day would give you five micrograms. Supermarkets and health food stores now provide several grain products fortified with added Vitamin B-12. Nutrigrain and GrapeNuts cereal have fortified their wheat and corn flakes, so one to two cups would meet all your B-12 requirements. Tempeh miso (fermented soybean) and tamari are both fermented by bacteria that manufacture sufficient B-12. Other non-animal sources of B-12 include the algae, spirulina and seaweed with bacteria clinging to its surface.

RDA: 4 mcg.
Supplement pills contain breakdown of B-12 and are not used as efficiently as the whole foods listed

below. Friendly microorganisms (algae, bacteria) provide the ideal source of B-12 between 4 to 25 mcg./day. If the "intrinsic factor" enzyme (produced by your body) is absent, your body would not absorb this vitamin properly. The doctor may decide you need injections of B-12. Fortunately, this deficiency is rare. No toxicity has been reported by overdose.

1 CUP or 2 oz. as noted	mcg.
Plankton - spirulina	160.00
Dried seaweeds	1.6 - 100
Oysters, 2 oz.	10.20
Crab, 2 oz.	5.70
Herring, 2 oz.	5.10
Nutritional yeast, 2 tbls.	4.00
Nutri-Grain wheat/corn cereal	3.00
Grape-Nuts cereal, w/B-12	1.50
Flank steak, 2 oz.	.68
Chicken broth	.24
Miso (fermented soybean)	.17

VITAMIN B-1

Vitamin B-1, thiamine, has been discovered to be very essential to good health. If you do not get enough B-1, it can lead to fatigue, loss of appetite, emotional problems, beriberi, excess hyperthyroidism, shingles and in severe cases - death. The RDA for Vitamin B-1 is set at 1 to 1.8 milligrams. It's important to take the B-1 as a complex, if you do use it as a supplement. A supplement range could be safe from two to one hundred milligrams per day. The higher dosage would be taken if you consume large amounts of alcohol or sugars. The lower dosage of two milligrams would be used as a preventive formula in combination with the other B complex vitamins.

To get proper B-1 from your foods, you could use sprouted sunflower seeds. Just one cup per day meets your entire Vitamin B-1 requirement. Millet, split peas, green peas, bulgur wheat, asparagus and brown rice are all good sources of B-1. B-1 deficiencies occur when people eat large amount of processed foods, such as white bread, white rice, sugars and alcohol. Because there is not enough Vitamin B-1 in processed white flour and sugar to metabolize all the carbohydrates. It's best to switch to whole natural foods, such as whole wheat bread with all its B Vitamins intact instead of white bread.

RDA: 1 - 1.8 mg.

Supplement must be taken as a B complex (with other B's) in range from 2 to 100 mg./day. The better your diet, the less you need supplements. The more processed white flours, sugar or alcohol you use, the higher the dosage of B's.

1 CUP or as noted	mg.
Sprouted sunflower seeds	2.84
Millet	1.66
Split peas	1.48
Black beans	1.10
Green peas	.51
Bulgur wheat	.48
Asparagus	.24
Red kidney or pinto beans	.20
Oatmeal, old fashioned	.19
Sunflower seeds, 1/4 cup	.18
Brown rice	.18
Mung bean sprouts	.14

VITAMIN B-2 RIBOFLAVIN

Riboflavin is essential to good health, but it's the most common deficiency Americans develop. The RDA has been set at 1.4 to 2 milligrams. To meet your needs, include the following foods that are good sources of B-2: wild rice, millet, mushrooms, collards, broccoli, various beans and peas. Deficiencies can occur, and they may show up as cracks in the corners of your mouth and childrens growth also can be affected.

RDA: 1.4 - 2 mg.
B-2 is the most common American deficiency. Supplement range 2 to 100 mg./day.

1 CUP	mg.
Wild rice	1.01
Millet	.87
Mushrooms	.32
Broccoli	.31
Collards	.29
Winter squash	.27
Alfalfa sprouts	.21
Split peas	.18
Pinto or black beans	.13
Pumpkin	.12
Whole wheat bread (3 slices)	.06

VITAMIN B-3

The RDA for niacin, Vitamin B-3, has been established between 15-20 milligrams. 1 1/2 cups of broccoli would meet all your requirements for the day. Sprouted sunflower seeds, split peas, mushrooms and beans are all good sources.

If you develop a deficiency of B-3 it can lead to pellagra, a condition in which the skin develops small spots that look like dirt or suntan. It can lead to paralysis and death. But, you can get too much niacin and excesses above 1,000 milligrams per day have been known to cause headache, liver damage and possible blindness. Time-released Niacinamide has been shown to be safer, however, don't exceed our recommended dosages. To obtain good results, the safe supplement range would be between 20 -100 milligrams per day. Any dose beyond this should be under the care and direction of a physician.

RDA: 15 - 20 mg.

Niacin deficiency may cause depression, insomnia or pellagra (dermititis, diarrhea, etc.). A safe supplement range is 20 to 100 mg. per day. Over 200 mg. of niacin may harm the delicate blood vessels in the eye due to excessive dilation. Niacinamide does not have this effect; but, dosages of 2,000 mg. may cause liver damage, depression and gout. Food is your best source, with supplements in moderation.

1 CUP	**mg.**
Broccoli	9.7
Sprouted sunflower seeds	9.0
Wholemeal flour	8.3
Split peas	7.0
Soybeans	6.1
Mushroooms	5.7
Beans, (pinto, black, etc.)	4.2
Oats	3.3
Wholemeal bread	1.8

VITAMIN B-6

This vitamin is called pyridoxine and the RDA is set at two milligrams. It is needed to metabolize amino acids and for the formation of hemoglobin in red blood cells. If you eat two cups of brown rice per day, this would meet your B-6 requirements. Bananas are also a good source, as are chestnuts, one of the few nuts low in fat.

RDA: 2 mg.

Safe supplement range 2 to 25 mg. Deficiency symptoms are similar to niacin and riboflavin deficiencies - muscular weakness, depression, cracks around mouth and eyes, etc.

1 CUP	mg.
Brown rice	1.00
Banana (1)	.76
Chestnuts	.53
Carrot juice	.50
Corn	.47

FOLIC ACID

This is another important member of the B complex family. The RDA is set at 400 micrograms and if you take a folic acid supplement, we suggest you include it as part of a B complex. One of the best sources would be boysenberries. A cup would meet nearly one-fourth of your daily need. Oranges, strawberries, tangerines, pears and rhubarb are other sources.

RDA: 400 mcg. (.4 mg.)

Supplement in B complex up to 400 mcg.

1 CUP	**mcg.**
Boysenberries	83.60
Cantaloupe, 1/2 melon	45.50
Orange	39.70
Avocado, 1/4	31.00
Strawberries	26.40
Black beans	24.70
Tangerine	17.10
Pear, 1	12.10
Rhubarb	8.70

PANTOTHENIC ACID

Another of the B complex, the RDA is five to ten milligrams. Good sources of pantothenic acid are mushrooms, brown rice, hot red chili peppers, cabbage, cauliflower and wheat bran. Sunflower seeds when sprouted are another source. If you take a supplement, a safe range would be five to thirty milligrams.

RDA: 5 to 10 mg.

Supplement range 5 to 30 mg.

1 CUP	**mg.**
Hot red chili pepper	2.60
Brown rice	2.10
Sunflower seeds, sprouted	2.00
Cauliflower	1.60
Wheat bran	1.60
Mushrooms	1.54
Cabbage	1.14
Pomegranate	1.00
Chestnuts	.76
Corn	.73
Oatmeal, cooked	.50

VITAMIN C

The RDA for this vitamin is 60 milligrams and you could get this amount from one orange. You might not be aware strawberries have twice the Vitamin C as oranges, broccoli has three times more, red peppers have four times as much and red, hot chili peppers have seven times as much more Vitamin C per cup quantity.

Remember, to get the most Vitamin C, it's always best to eat these foods as fresh as possible, either when they come from the tree or fresh from your sprouting jar. If you take a supplement, the range would be from 60-500 milligrams per day. In certain instances you may have been advised to take more than 1,000 milligrams by your physician, and if so, you should follow those guidelines.

You can store Vitamin C in your white blood cell buffycoat. Most people can saturate their storage capacity, if they get at least 100 milligrams of Vitamin C per day. A lack of Vitamin C usually only occurs if you're deprived of fruits and vegetables or in a more serious situation of starvation. This lack of Vitamin C can lead to scurvy - bleeding gums, sores, loose teeth, swollen legs and possible death. Again, all fresh fruits and vegetables will supply you with a good source of Vitamin C.

RDA: 60 mg.

Supplement range 50-500 mg.

1 CUP	mg.
Hot red chili peppers	369
Guavas, 1 medium	242
Red sweet peppers	204
Black currants	200
Broccoli	140
Turnip greens	139
Brussels sprouts	135
Kale	125
Green peppers	102
Collards	92
Kiwi fruit	89
Strawberries	85
Cauliflower	78
Red cabbage	61
Orange	50
Asparagus	45

VITAMIN D

The RDA is established at 400 I.U.; a safe supplement range would be up to 400 I.U. It would be best not to exceed this amount, because too much Vitamin D could lead to a type of calcification of the arteries. In England this overdose side effect had been reported in infants. Now in that country, you can only get Vitamin D by prescription.

Your best source of Vitamin D is the sunlight. By stepping outdoors for 15 minutes, you will allow your body to produce all the Vitamin D it requires. It may be a cloudy day, but if part of your face and skin are exposed, you'll produce Vitamin D.

RDA: 400 I.U.

Supplement range under 400 I.U. 15 minutes outdoors in daylight allows your body to produce all the required Vitamin D. If climate or clothing does not permit this, a growing child would need a supplement or 3 oz. of fish per day.

ZINC

Good sources of this mineral are garbanzo beans, whole wheat flour, wheat bran, lentil and soybean sprouts. A supplement between 15-25 milligrams is a reasonable amount.

RDA: 15 to 25 mg.
Same for supplement range.

1 CUP	mg.
Wheat bran	5.60
Garbanzos	5.40
Whole wheat flour	2.90
Soy sprouts	1.70
Lentil sprouts	1.70

SELENIUM

The amount of selenium in food varies depending on the concentration in soil where it was grown. The basic RDA is .05 to 2 milligrams. Onions, cabbage, carrots, potatoes, tomatoes, grains, cereals, fruits and vegetables are all sources of selenium. The Delgado Health Plan is higher in selenium than most typical diets.

Some studies seem to suggest selenium reduces the risk of heart disease. Of course, people eating the most selenium were also eating more whole grains, fruits and vegetables, and as we already know, these foods are low in fat and cholesterol. As a result, it's not clear if selenium is the main factor in lowering the risk of heart disease. But, selenium is an anti-oxidant and can help improve and maintain good health by reducing the effects of processed foods.

RDA: 50 mcg./day (.05 to .20 mg./day)

Supplement range 50 to 100 mcg. per day (.05 to .10 mg.). Toxic at 5,000 mcg. (5 mg./day) long-term use. Foods vary greatly in concentration of selenium; depends on the amount present in the soil in which it was grown.

SERVING	Lowest to highest in mcg.
Onion, raw (1/2 cup)	1.3 (MD) to 1,513 (SD)*
Cabbage, 1/2 cup	1.8 (MD) to 316 (SD)
Carrot, raw (1)	1.8 (MD) to 105 (SD)
Potato, raw (1)	1.0 (MD) to 235 (SD)
Tomatoes, 2 medium	1.4 (MD) to 329 (SD)
Grains/cereals	Average 12.3
Fruits/vegetables	Average .9 to 1.6
Seafood/chicken (2 oz.)	Average 12 to 16

* MD (Maryland) SD (South Dakota)

IRON

The RDA's for iron are 10 milligrams for men and 18 for women. The supplement amount also should stay in this range. Iron is needed to produce hemoglobin in the blood to carry oxygen and to prevent anemia, pallor and fatigue. Dairy products frequently cause iron-deficiency anemia by inhibiting iron absorption (American Journal of Clinical Nutrition 33:86, 1988). If this problem develops, stop drinking cow's milk.

Too much iron can cause toxic side effects. For example, an intake of over 200 milligrams per day has been known to lead to liver disorders. If you took in 3 to 20 grams per day it could lead to iron overload of the liver and possible death. The Bantu natives who do all their cooking in iron pots, have a tremendous iron toxicity problem because excess iron gets into their food. Iron overload kills more people, percentage-wise, in this culture than heart disease does in our country. If you are cooking with iron pots every day, I would suggest you alternate with other types of cookware.

Good sources of iron include sprouted sunflower seeds, garbanzo beans, lentils, parsley, split peas and seaweed.

RDA: 10 mg. for male, 18 mg. for female.

Supplement range 10 to 18 mg./day. Toxic side effects over 200 mg./day.

1 CUP	**mg.**
Hijiki, seaweed	29.00
Wheat bran	14.70
Tomato paste	9.20
Sunflower seeds, sprouted	7.70
Garbanzo beans	6.70
Tofu, soybean curd	5.20
Kidney beans, cooked	4.40
Lentils, cooked	4.20
Parsley	3.70
Split peas, cooked	3.40
Beet greens	3.30

CALCIUM

Calcium is essential to good bone integrity, to maintaining strong healthy teeth and for proper nerve and muscle functioning. The RDA has been established at 800 to 1,200 milligrams. This range can be easily met by eating a variety of foods, including turnip greens, collards, kale, cabbage, garbanzo beans, broccoli and corn tortillas. There is more calcium in five tortillas than in a cup of milk.

Milk is not a safe source of calcium because some people cannot tolerate the use of dairy products. Many races have an allergic reaction; the production of a certain enzyme is inhibited and the dairy products remain undigested. Some symptoms of this intolerance include diarrhea, disorientation, bloating or distending of the stomach due to the milk or dairy products rotting in the stomach.

You get more calcium, ounce per ounce, from vegetables and various beans and peas. Although the Dairy Council says you must drink milk every day and use dairy products regularly to get your RDA of calcium, this is not true. When you reduce your protein intake and increase the intake of complex carbohydrates, your body will absorb calcium much more efficiently.

Yet, if your protein intake is high, you may develop bone-related problems. For example, the Eskimos consume about 2,000 milligrams of calcium per day, they even eat the bones of the fish they catch! Surprisingly, they develop osteoporosis, loss of bone material, fractures and weakened bones, all by the age of 40. How can this be? The Eskimos' diet is 25% protein.

If you exceed 15% of your calories in protein, it leaves acid or waste product in the blood. As a result, minerals like calcium, magnesium and zinc are drawn right out of the bones to neutralize the excess acid, to maintain the PH of the blood. The penalty, though, is weakening of the bones, loss of teeth and an increased rate of fracture, which happens in our culture so frequently. Hip fractures have recently been considered the major cause of death in women past the age of 50. It has even surpassed the death rate from breast cancer. Once a person is debilitated from this fracture and bed-ridden, they may develop infections, pneumonia and other problems that lead to death.

Osteoporosis can be offset simply by reducing your protein intake and eating whole, natural foods. Ironically, some people try to increase their calcium intake by eating more dairy products. If you do, you'll probably get too much protein and untimately lose more calcium from the bones. According to the American Journal of Clinical Nutrition (Volume 41, 1985) women with osteoporosis were divided into two groups. Half were asked to drink three glasses of milk per day and the other half had none. After one year, the women drinking milk lost more calcium out of their bones than the women avoiding milk. Ironically, this study was sponsored by the National Dairy Council, and it showed the overconsumption of protein from milk offset the increase of 1,500 mg. of calcium in the milk.

The U.S. and Finland have the highest milk and protein intake in the world (90-100 g. per day) and the greatest number of hip fractures. Hong Kong and South Africa (black townships) have the lowest number of hip fractures - they consume the least milk and less than 80 grams of protein per day. Studies have shown if the protein intake is over 90 grams per day, the acid build-up in the blood will cause you to excrete more calcium through the urine than you can possibly take in, even if you take supplements. This loss of calcium and other minerals from the body is known as negative mineral inbalance.

Further studies of the Bantu natives in South Africa provide us with important information regarding calcium. The Bantu women give birth to an average of nine children and nurse each child an average of two years. You would assume these women need large amounts of calcium since they spend eighteen years lactating. But, their average diet contains only 350 milligrams of calcium a day. They eat mostly complex carbohydrates, whole grains, some vegetables and fruit, about a 10% protein diet. Because of this low-protein diet they have no calcium deficiencies, they have strong bones, they don't lose their teeth as they get older, their children grow up healthy and free of rickets and the other calcium deficiency problems that occur in other cultures. Osteoporosis, which occurs so frequently in our culture, is non-existent in the Bantu culture.

How do they do it? Their diet is a well-balanced, nutritious combination of whole grains, fruits and vegetables, without the excess use of protein. The calcium they eat is absorbed properly and they maintain good health. Studies on people who eat grains, vegetables and fruit and avoid meat and dairy products have shown they have stronger bone density on x-ray than do meat-eaters.

We know osteoporosis can be conquered now simply by changing the diet and exercising regularly. We know exercise increases calcium absorption in the bones and we have found aerobic exercises help to retain calcium. If you smoke, you should know smoking pulls calcium out of the bones and pushes it into the soft tissues of the arteries. Finally, if you're taking a supplement, stay in the 300-800 milligram range per day and it should be taken in a 1 to-1 balance with magnesium.

RDA: 800 to 1,400 mg.

Supplement range 300 to 800 mg., to be taken in 2 to 1 balance with magnesium. Be sure to avoid excess protein which depletes calcium.

1 CUP	**mg.**
Sesame seeds, unhulled *	1,740
Seaweed	1,000
Corn tortillas, 5	310
Nonfat milk	302
Turnip greens	267
Collards	220
Kale	206
Cabbage	165
Garbanzo beans	150
Pinto beans	150
Broccoli	136
Parsley	122
Oranges	119
Rhubarb	105
Navy beans	95
Rutabaga	92
Human milk	80

* 1 tbsp. of sesame seeds has 93 mg. of calcium (more than 1 cup of human milk) and only 2.6 grams fat and 30 calories. Sesame seeds that have been hulled (outer seed coat removed) have lost 90% of the calcium.

POTASSIUM

We need about 2,500 milligrams of potassium per day. The first thing many people say is, "I eat bananas." Of course, bananas are a good source of potassium, but did you know garbanzo beans are three times higher in potassium? Winter squash is also higher, and tomatoes are as high in potassium as bananas. Cantaloupes, carrots, avocados and potatoes are all good sources, too.

RDA: 2,500 mg.

Fruits and vegetables are the best source.

1 CUP or as noted	mg.
Split peas	1,790
Garbanzo beans	1,584
Lima beans	1,162
Winter squash	946
Tomato, 2 medium	888
Banana, 2 medium	880
Potato, 1 medium	782
Peach, 2 medium	616

Cantaloupe, 1/4 melon	341
Avocado, 1/4	340
Carrot, 1	246

MAGNESIUM

RDA: 300 to 450 mg.

Magnesium helps to relax the muscles after calcium stimulates contraction of muscles. Magnesium helps to regulate body temperature, acid-base balance and the absorption and use of other minerals. Small amounts of magnesium appear to help people with chronic insomnia, muscle cramps, headaches, depression and irregular heart rhythm. High blood cholesterol levels, high protein diets, diuretics or alcoholism creates an increased need for magnesium.

1 CUP or as noted	mg.
Millet, dry	369
Whole wheat flour	136
Beet greens	106
Swiss chard	97
Almonds (1/4 cup)	95
Black eyed peas, cooked	90
Collards	84
Whole wheat rolls, 2	80
Potato, baked (1)	75
Yam	62
Oatmeal, cooked	56

Kohlrabi	55
Green peas	50
Spinach	44
Prunes	38
Whole wheat bread (2 slices)	36
Banana (1)	33
Corn tortilla (1)	32
Cantaloupe (1/2)	28
Tomato (1 medium)	21
Summer squash	21

FAT (LINOLEIC ACID)

Requirement: 1% of total calories; i.e.,: you need 2.22 grams of linoleic acid fat on a 2,000 calorie diet. Avoid oils and separate fats. Whole food is your best source of fat (see below).

SERVING	grams
Sunflower seeds, 1/4 cup	2.90
Walnuts, 1/4 oz.	2.80
Oatmeal, 2 cups	2.00
Sesame seeds, 1 tbsp.	1.80
Avocado, 1/4	1.20
Chicken breast, 1/2	1.10
Whole wheat bread, 2 slices	.40
Popcorn, 2 cups plain	.40
Lettuce	(varies)

PROTEIN

Requirement: 40 grams per day (up to a maximum of 74 grams). Eat enough calories to meet your ideal body weight, with complex carbohydrates to spare protein. Whole grains are one of the best sources of balanced proteins and are ideally suited for human needs according to recent studies. *

SERVING	grams
Split peas, 1 cup	16.00
Navy beans, 1 cup	15.00
Black-eyed peas, 1 cup	13.40
Flank steak, 2 oz.	12.00
Halibut, 2 oz.	11.90
Scallops, 2 oz.	8.70
Lentil sprouts, 1 cup	8.40
Collards, 1 cup	6.80
Brussels sprouts, 1 cup	6.50
Soybean sprouts, 1 cup	6.50
Oatmeal, 1 cup	6.00
Green peas, 1 cup	5.90
Alfalfa sprouts, 1 cup	5.10
Kale, 1 cup	5.00
Shredded wheat, 1 cup	5.00
Brown rice, 1 cup	4.90
Yams, 1 cup	4.80
Asparagus, 1 cup	3.40
Cherries, 1 cup	1.74

NOTE:

1. Nuts contain an unprocessed fat with fiber that slows the absorption, while providing a significant source of nutrients. However, nuts are concentrated in calories and fat, so limit their intake.

2. Seeds can be sprouted, which reduces their fat content to an ideal low-fat level.

3. Animal products should be eaten in amounts not exceeding (per day) 3 oz. of lean meat, 2 glasses of nonfat milk and 1 cup of nonfat yogurt. (Avoidance of all dairy products and meats would be ideal for nutritional considerations). Reducing protein use will help to prevent dehydration, fatigue and loss of calcium, magnesium, zinc, etc. from your bones.

4. Eat a variety of whole grains (at least 2 different types per day), vegetables, fruits, beans, peas, nuts, seeds and sprouts.

SAFE SUPPLEMENTAL RANGE (per day)

VITAMINS

Beta-Carotene A	5,000 to 10,000 I.U.
B-12	4 to 24 mcg.
B-1	2 to 100 mcg.
B-2	2 to 100 mcg.
B-3	15 to 100 mcg.
B-6	2 to 25 mg.
Folic Acid	100 to 400 mcg.
Pantothenic Acid	5 to 30 mg.
C	50 to 500 mg.
D	50 to 400 I.U.
E	10 to 400 I.U.

MINERALS

Calcium	300 to 800 mg.
Magnesium	200 to 450 mg.
Iron	10 to 18 mg.
Potassium	800 to 2500 mg.
Selenium	50 to 100 mcg.
Zinc	15 to 25 mg.
Linoleic acid (1% of total calories)	2 to 4 grams
Protein	30 to 74 grams
Carbohydrate	300 to 400 grams

STORING VITAMINS AND MINERALS

Don't worry if you can't eat all the foods I have suggested. By eating a variety and alternating the foods you eat from day to day, you won't have to worry about deficiencies because your body has a storage capacity. For example, your body can store potassium for one to two days, if you aren't getting any new source of potassium. You can store calcium from ten to twenty years, in the bones especially. Of course, you don't want to deplete your calcium, otherwise later, the penalty will be weakened bones. Understand, though you don't have to take in a calcium source every day. The foods we recommend have an ability to provide you with enough calcium. This is supported by recent studies that show calcium is absorbed just as well by these foods as from other sources. Iron can be stored for four to five months. Vitamin A is stored from one to two years. Vitamin B-12 is stored from ten to twenty and Vitamin B-3 has a storage of two to three months.

Sodium can be stored about two to three days and the problem here is excessive sodium intake. Your body needs about one to two grams per day. We get all we need from whole natural foods. If you eat packaged foods that have sodium added, you'll probably add another one to two grams a day, but this is still a low-sodium diet. If you add salt to your food, you'll push it up to ten grams or more and then you will retain fluid and have other side effects. Also, you don't need to add sodium to your diet when you're exercising more. The body will adapt and adjust itself to conserve sodium as necessary, even if the temperature is very warm.

Water can be stored for about four days, and interestingly enough, has been recently shown to affect your endurance levels. It was found if athletes were deprived of water before exercising, they would fatigue much quicker. If they were allowed to drink extra water before and during the exercise, they lasted the longest. A third group of athletes, who could only drink water after they started when they were thirsty, lasted an intermediate amount of time. We have found now it's best to hydrate yourself before exercise. The rule of thumb is drink about a cup for every 15 minutes of intense exercise activity you anticipate and another cup for every 50 pounds of body weight. For example, if you weigh 150 pounds, drink three cups for body weight, and another two cups if you plan to exercise for thirty minutes. Those five cups may seem like a large amount, but you can function at your maximum intensity that day during exercise, especially if it's hot outside.

Carbohydrates can only be stored for a few hours. This is important to know because if you don't eat frequent small meals, your blood sugar level may drop and then you have a hypoglycemic reaction. You'll be fatigued and tired, and then it's hard to get the glucose back to a good range. It's helpful to eat regular amounts of potatoes, grains, fruits and vegetables to maintain that glucose level. On our plan you may notice you'll eat more often because you have less fat in your diet. Fat sits in your stomach and has so many calories it takes away your appetite. Complex carbohydrates are burned efficiently and cleanly. Instead of eating three meals, you'll be eating four or five. It's okay to eat between meals and you should plan each day to do so if you want constant energy.

We store protein about six to seven weeks. We get a good source of protein with all the necessary amino acids from our whole natural foods. Fat is stored six to seven weeks. Some people tell me they store it longer than six or seven weeks and when you look at them, it's hard not to agree!!

ENEMIES TO GOOD NUTRITION

Some enemies to vitamin and mineral nutrition would be: white sugar, white rice, white flour, alcohol, cigarettes, antacids (they deplete various minerals) and baking soda (depletes the B vitamins). Unfortunately, in our society, some of these products will slip into our diet, so you probably will need some kind of supplement for preventive reasons.

There are also hidden additives in foods. Ice cream, for example, contains Diethyl Glucol, which is also used in anti-freeze and paint removers. A vanilla substitute, Piperonal, is also used to exterminate lice. A certain cherry flavoring (Alydehyde C 17) is used in rubber dyes and plastic; pineapple flavoring (Ethyl Acetate) is used to clean textiles and leather. There is a nut flavoring (Butradlehyde) used in rubber cement, a banana flavoring (Amyl Acetate) used in paint solvent - the list seems endless. Why don't they tell you these common food additives are solvents and are used in these products? It's because the food manufacturers aren't required by law to put the original name on the labels; they can simply say "banana flavoring" instead of its true name: Amyl Acetate. So, just because these names aren't labeled on your foods, it doesn't mean the foods are healthy for you. It's best to stick with whole, natural foods.

We also have to contend with the inevitable environmental pollution. In studies conducted by

Cal-Tech, it was found we have a 500% increase of lead in our bodies, compared with prehistoric man. It only takes four times than that to reach a toxic level. We are at a borderline now that is why there has been a movement toward unleaded gasoline and getting lead out of paint bases and so forth. These heavy metals can build up in our bodies. According to the medical journal, Lancet, certain tests like hair analysis, can access the amount of toxic metals in the body. There are certain foods that can help remove these heavy metals. Foods high in soluble fibers, such as beans, peas, apples, pears, oat bran and corn flakes, seem to stick to heavy metals and reduce their content in the body. These foods also lower cholesterol, so you should use them as a preventive formula.

FAT REQUIREMENTS

What about fat intake? You do need fat in the diet. Linoleic acid is considered an essential fatty acid. You only need about 2% of your total calories in linoleic acid, which is about two to four grams. You should not add oils or fats to your diet to get linoleic acid, because they are processed, and ironically, when you add oils to your diet it can deplete the linoleic acid and cause fat deficiency. Your best source of linoleic acid would be natural foods, such as whole sunflower sprouts and oatmeal. Two cups of oatmeal will give you all the linoleic acid you need. Two or three walnuts, five or six almonds or a tablespoon of sesame seeds are all good sources. Lettuce and small amounts of avocado are also great sources of linoleic acid.

Don't use processed oils to get your fat supply. To make corn or sunflower oils, for example, a solvent is first poured on the kernels or seeds. It is then heated to a very high temperature, and lye and bleaching agents are added. Odors are produced, so they add an antioxidant. As a result, a residual solvent is left in the oil, and then this is called "purified oil." Cold processed oil is no better; the only step they omit is the heating process.

You would not think of sugar as a good source of food. Yet sugar was processed from the whole sugar beet, and sugar beets are perfectly healthy for you. The same is true of corn oil; corn is healthy, but if you extract the oil, it's processed and loses its beneficial qualities.

If you must use oil in your diet, for cooking and recipes, rely on a very small amount of olive oil. It has a strong flavor and extends a long way, so you can use a much smaller amount. In cooking you can use non-stick pans or the microwave.

Now that you have an understanding of vitamins, minerals, protein and fat, you also may be interested in what kind of supplements to take. There are so many different products and name brands. I suggest you look at the vitamin and mineral labels. Read the dosages, the amount of each nutrient and see if they match the ranges we recommend. You want to make sure you get enough, but remember too much can cause toxic side effects that are harmful. Always begin with whole natural foods, then check to see if your supplement falls into the proper range. If you find extra sugar or alcohol slipping into your diet, be sure to use the higher end of the ranges for the B complex vitamins.

Study the following section to put together a winning combination for you and your family. Identify the foods you currently eat and see if they are listed in each category for vitamins and minerals. If you haven't used supplements before, purchase those that fall into the safe supplement range.

VITAMIN-RICH FOODS AND THE SAFE SUPPLEMENT RANGE

Good food sources of vitamins and minerals are those that have the richest content. All whole natural foods that are unprocessed and eaten fresh are excellent sources of vitamins and minerals. Learning which foods to eat and making a variety of selections will give you a better chance of obtaining ideal health.

Certain foods (liver, egg yolks, cheese, etc.) were not listed because they are too high in such harmful substances as fat, cholesterol and salt. You would be smart to eat the other foods that are safe to eat, even in large amounts.

Supplements may be used as a preventive measure (especially if you occasionally drink alcohol or use processed foods, white flour or sugar). The daily intake should include vitamins and minerals based on the complete ranges listed in this section. While the RDA's are also listed to help you, our safe ranges are based on medical research reports of deficiency from sub-optimal levels and on toxicity from overuse of supplements. Compare your supplement brands for best results.

* For more information on protein requirements, please see Nick Delgado's book "Weight Loss and Energy Now".

CHAPTER EIGHTEEN

SEX

Some common sexual problems identified by the Archives of Internal Medicine, March 1981, are consistently due to the following two factors: diabetes, a well-known cause of male impotency and coronary heart disease - patients frequently shun or avoid sexual activities because of the pervasive fear of sudden cardiac death. We have all heard of individuals who died during sexual activity, so naturally people with angina or chest pains are afraid of this situation.

Impotency also can be caused by long-term use of antihypertensive drugs (high blood pressure medications) because blood flow is reduced to the male organ so much there isn't enough blood to achieve an erection. We also know shortness of breath can lead to sexual problems. If you are not in good physical shape at that critical point, you may fall short of complete enjoyment.

Masters and Johnson, who originally went on record to say most sexual problems were due to mental fears, have now completely changed their original opinion. They now believe most cases of sexual problems or inadequacy are caused by degenerative-type diseases. As we know, cholesterol often begins filling up blood vessels and closing off the arteries leading to the sexual organs. If this happens, there is a deadening of feeling and a loss of function. Thirty-four percent of middle-aged men suffer from impotence, with most cases caused from poor circulation.

We have seen men who were sexually impotent reverse this problem because of improved blood flow throughout the body due to dietary changes. Because of this improvement, medications were discontinued. The reduction of fat and cholesterol in the diet can restore blood flow to the penis and by improving the circulation, angina and chest pains are also eliminated.

I will ask if you are physically fit. One of the best preparations is to start a walking or jogging program. Of course, you also must begin a dietary approach so you can begin to look more physically attractive and internally healthy. Begin doing sit-up exercises because during sexual activity, much emphasis is placed on the abdominal area. As you become more physically fit, you will become more attractive, which will result in building your confidence and leads to an improved sex life.

Do you T.C.K.? Can you guess what these initials represent? Touch, Caress, Kiss. If you touch, caress and kiss for at least 20 minutes this will build intensity to continue an extremely pleasant activity.

It is important to build intensity for greater sexual response. "The Hite Report" was probably the most thorough report of both male and female sexuality. Other reference book include "Women and Sex in the 80's - the Cosmo Report", by Linda Wolf, "Shared Intimacies" by Linda Levine, A.C.S.W. and Lonnie Barbach, Ph.D.; "The Intimate Male, candid discussions about women, sex and relationships" by Linda Levine and Lonnie Barbach and "The Ultimate Pleasure, The secrets of easily orgasmic women" by Marc and Judith Meshorer. These books will increase your knowledge of human sexuality and present you with important information.

In summary (from The Hite Report), less than 30% of women achieve an orgasm by intercourse. This is not so surprising when we understand that for years women were discouraged from enjoying direct clitoral stimulation. This was considered an immature form of sexual orgasm as compared to those orgasms reached by intercourse (male researchers promoted this self-serving belief). However, physiologically, the clitoris is not located in a position where stimulation is easily reached during intercourse.

The best book written on the subject of sex from a Christians' perspective is "The Christian Guide to Sexual Fulfillment, Gift of Sex", by Clifford and Joyce Penner, published by World Book; Waco, Texas. The Bible gives us an understanding about the natural acts of masturbation and heterosexual behavior. The book by the Penners explains how a vibrator can be used to guide a woman to understand her own sexual response (the Hitachi plug-in model works best). Clitoral stimulation can be accomplished by manual manipulation and by oral sex. This removes pressure from the man to "perform" to bring a woman to orgasm by intercourse. Since women rarely achieve orgasm from intercourse, there is an uncomfortable pressure brought into the relationship. This pressure is relieved by a better understanding of human sexual response. The man and woman must understand that good sex is not determined by how long a man can last during intercourse. The techniques of the correct pressure and sensation directed at the female sites of pleasure can and must be learned and shared together.

Another interesting reference book, The G Spot, by Alice Kahn Ladas, Beverly Whipple and John D. Perry, has brought sexual psychology to a new brink of exciting knowledge. The G Spot, named after a physician named Grafenberg who discovered it in

1950, often leads to orgasms in women other than the commonly known clitoral orgasm. For three years, two researchers have been steadily building sizable evidence that suggests the following:

1. There is a sexual organ in women that is called the G spot.
2. Rubbing the G spot can lead to multiple and deeper orgasms more easily.
3. Women may expel fluid (ejaculate) from their vaginas when they have a G spot orgasm.

It is still important the male satisfy the female first by direct stimulation of the clitoris or by massaging the G spot. Let your imagination consider how this can be done, or even better, conduct your own research by investing in the excellent reference books mentioned above.

Many people have wondered if as they become older, will they still enjoy sex? According to Masters and Johnson, the record for multiple orgasms (under laboratory conditions) was held by a woman 70 years old. She had over fifty with the assistance of a vibrator. After eight hours, the researchers had to push her out the door, although she did have a smile on her face! At any rate, we do not know what the ultimate is in human capability.

A women's sexual desire can increase at menopause because of the hormone testosterone. This hormone, which enhances sexual desire, is produced by the adrenal glands at an accelerated rate and begins to dominate the estrogen. This is why many women report more sexual interest, pleasure and capacity for orgasm at this time.

According to a recent study, male menopause does not seem to occur, because there is no change in the sex hormone levels. Men can maintain erection longer, with more time between orgasms. This change in response can match the need of women who take longer to lubricate because of age. More time for imaginative, tender lovemaking would be ideal for both sexes.

CHAPTER NINETEEN

MENOPAUSE AND PMS

Urinary incontinence can occur from a weak PC (pubococcygeus) muscle. The "love muscle" is exercised by sexual intercourse or by squeezing the vagina as though trying to stop the flow of urine. It requires daily use - at least 200 contractions per day. Do 20 squeezes 10 times a day (at home, office, watching TV, etc.) Squeeze and relax the muscle as rapidly as you can and end with a long, sustained contraction. According to Dr. Kegel, these exercises have replaced the need for surgery in most women. It also helps to increase the intensity of orgasm. Men can also exercise their PC muscle and improve the pleasure and sensitivity of their orgasm.

Women are using powerful hormone replacement therapy pills prescribed by doctors and P.M.S. clinics with little regard to the potential long-term serious side effects. These hormone pills increase the risk of cancer and blood clotting. Fortunately, there is an alternative, safe course to follow using diet and exercise. The claim that hormone pills prevent osteoporosis is not completely true. Evidence showing the slowing of bone loss has been documented. However, there is a better way to prevent bone loss and strengthen the bone. Osteoporosis is caused by high protein diet and lack of sufficient exercise. If you start a daily walking program today, with weight training two times a week, you can immediately replace lost bone material. The high complex carbohydrate diet centers meals around grains, vegetables and fruit, instead of around proteins like meat, fish, chicken, milk and cheese. As you follow this lower protein diet your bones will begin to reabsorb lost bone material. You will receive adequate protein from the carbohydrate foods.

Before and after x-rays of people with osteoporosis has demonstrated a strengthening of bones by reducing dietary protein and exercising daily. Urine tests measuring calcium retention have shown immediate improvements of positive calcium balance (more calcium has been absorbed than lost). People on a high protein diet who do not exercise lose more calcium out of the urine than they take in from their diet. Hormone pills are not the answer - diet and exercise are the key to building bones with age.

Women are told to use hormones for mood changes of depression and irritability just before the menstrual cycles (Premenstrual syndrome) and after menopause. Fat in the diet will cause hormonal imbalances. These drastic hormonal imbalances can be corrected by following our lowfat diet and by daily, long distance walking exercises. Hormones tend to cause weight gain by increasing fat production and increasing fluid retention. The Delgado Diet will help by reducing fluid retention and reducing body fat from the hips, thighs and stomach. You will look and feel great each additional month that you closely adhere to the plan.

The Delgado lowfat diet and exercise plan will also decrease and prevent fibroid tumors, uterine cysts, endometrial thickening and "heavy" periods.

We have several women come to our Delgado Medical Clinic who have stopped taking those hormone pills and faithfully followed the Delgado Diet and Exercise Plan with great success. These women report less fatigue, increased energy and control of mood swings. Many women have been able to avoid hysterectomy surgery as the pain caused by fibroid tumors and uterine cysts disappeared.

Menopausal women are told to use estrogen creams, estrogen patches and pills to keep the skin "beautiful and young". The following steps are safer and effective:

1. Avoid smoking. Smokers skin wrinkles 10 years sooner than non-smokers. Carbon monoxide deprives the skin in the face (near the smoke) of

oxygen. Look at a smoker and non-smokers face and you'll notice how many more wrinkles the smoker has.

2. Limit exposure to the sun and use the appropriate sun screens. The excess sun exposure ages and wrinkles the skin. A suntan gives your body a healthy look, but sun bathe only in the early morning or late afternoon for less than 1 hour to avoid overdosing from the sun.

3. DO NOT wash your skin with soap. Any kind of soap dries the skin because it contains sodium hydroxide. Sodium hydroxide is alkaline, which is also used in Drano toilet cleaners and used to remove grease. If you follow a lowfat diet you will not have oily skin. Therefore, you will not need soap on your face. You ask then, what should you use? A former Miss America used fresh, bottled water to rinse her face and body. Keep a bottle near the sink and in the shower. Use the bottled water as a final rinse. Your skin sloughs off old skin every three days. This is your bodys' way of cleansing itself. It would be acceptable to use soap under the arms, in the pelvic region and the hands to reduce bacteria and dirt exposure. Use a gentle shampoo, Ph balanced, with conditioner on the hair to avoid dry scalp.

Use lotions on your skin to prevent dryness. Your skin will radiate with health as you follow the Delgado lowfat diet. As your blood carries more oxygen, your skin will take on a youthful appearance without resorting to hormones.

There are successful, natural ways to adjust for the decrease of hormone production after menopause. The thinning of vaginal wall tissue can be solved by using vegetable or fruit oils such as coconut, apricot kernel, safflower, baby oil or Vitamin E oil. DON'T EAT THE OIL - Have your spouse apply it to the length of your vagina. K-Y Jelly can be used, but it may dry too quickly. Avoid oils containing alcohol, vaseline or petroleum jelly since they can cause infection or irritation.

Hot flashes can be reduced by exercise, which stimulates the ability to perspire and cools the body. The low-fat diet also may reduce symptoms and discomfort as your circulation improves. Consistent, vigorous exercise increases the circulation of both estrogen and adrenaline, toning the skin and muscles.

How to dramatically shrink your fat cells

Most people are born with too many fat cells. However, we discovered an amazing wa to dramatically shrink those fat cells down in size, so you'll look great!

Amazing way to reach your goal weight

Now you can reach your goal weight permanently by eating all day. Yes, that's righ just by consuming the foods that we teach you to eat, you will lose fat. You will get t choose the foods that you like to eat. **Imagine, you get to enjoy eating zesty Italian, flavorful Mexican and Chinese foods.**

Theresa Geske said, *"I can eat all the foods I want to eat as many times during the da as I would like. . . You're never feeling hungry."*

Have a beautiful body, radiant skin and hair

You will notice how much younger you look and feel after two weeks. Karen Reed Natural Ms. California 1991, excitedly noticed improvements, *"I'm always looking for th perfect diet plan. Something that would promote perfect health, help me to feel wonderful, los body fat and maintain muscle and I find that this plan has met all of my goals."*

You will have more energy

Participants say it's unlike anything they have ever experienced. **They wake-up alert they feel a sense of strength, and a consistent feeling of well-being.** Alexander Lord said,*"I improved my skin. It made my body look leaner. I have more energy. I require less sleep. .You will feel better than you've ever felt in your life."* And Moses Yim said, *"I've gotten younger physically and mentally. . .I'm 71 years old. . .I started to play golf again."*

Save money on wellness

Delgado plan participants report **an average savings of 15% every week on their grocer bills.** Karen Reed said, *"I'm saving at least $100 a month because I'm not using any of thos health food supplements I used to take."* Also, being well means not having to take pills You won't have to see the doctor except for wellness check-ins. Our doctors encourage you and applaude your progress. **You will be taking care of problems before they occur.** Mrs Lord said, *"You get your health back and you automatically spend less money on medical bills.* Your family will benefit more than they ever expected.

Call Delgado Medical today, (714) 540-7725 for an appointment to determine you needs and to begin the plan. Personal appointments, upcoming seminars, other events testing and educational materials are available to fit your needs.

DELGADO MEDICAL, 17150 NEWHOPE ST., SUITE 217
FOUNTAIN VALLEY, CALIFORNIA 92708

CHAPTER TWENTY

SUCCESS

To accomplish all the goals we have discussed, you need to be success oriented. You need to want success. To reach your goals be aware you may have what is called the "Fear of Success." Let me review some "Fear of Success" symptoms with you. If you can answer "yes" or if any of these statements pertain to you, you may have the "Fear of Success."

1. Do you believe good feelings can't last?
2. Do you dilute good times with reflections of past sadness or future catastrophes?
3. Is it easier to spend money on others than on yourself?
4. Are you afraid to leave a long-term job for a better offer?
5. Are you always late no matter how hard you try to be on time?
6. Do you have difficulty making decisions?
7. Are you a perfectionist? Do you fear making a mistake?
8. Do you procrastinate?
9. Are you detached to a fault, fearing intimacy or closeness?
10. Do you avoid relationships to eliminate the possibility of rejection?
11. Are you too shy to tell your partner what feels good to you?

12. Do you feel too fat for sex?
13. Is losing weight a losing battle for you?
14. When someone gives you a compliment, do you answer with negative statements?

If you feel any of these relate to you, then you may have what is called the "Fear of Success." The best way to overcome any of these problems is to start taking action and going after your needs. For instance, one of the most common problems that affects us is procrastination. You know there are certain projects you need to finish, yet you look at them and say you can always do it later. When you find yourself in that situation, repeat these words, "DO IT NOW!" You will be amazed how quickly you will begin to respond and start to work toward the toughest goals. You should make a special point of doing the tough jobs first. Late at night or early each morning I review tasks for the day and month. I assign them an order of priority in my Day Planner. Be efficient, every minute counts. Become organized, break big or important tasks down to small components. Complete them as quickly as possible and go on to the next task. Spend more time on those goals that will give you the biggest return. Procrastinate on those tasks which have little chance for reward. This is the key to proper time management. Use your time effectively and you will be successful.

One reason people are perfectionists is they are afraid to make mistakes. If you are a perfectionist and you have to make certain decisions, you should not be afraid of making mistakes. If you do make mistakes, be confident you can pick yourself up and recoup your forces.

If you have trouble losing weight, now is the time to make the affirmation you can reach this goal. The Delgado Health Plan works with you. Many people can become discouraged trying to lose weight after a couple of months because they have lost only 3 to 5 pounds. I worked with one woman who eventually lost 45 pounds. At the three month point, she was discouraged, though she had lost 20 pounds by that time. When she looked at herself, she didn't feel she had improved her shape as much as she wanted. We encouraged her to stick to her goals and keep applying our recommendations. She worked harder and is now enjoying the benefits. She has reshaped her body and looks like a new person. It also can work for you; just give yourself time.

If you fail at some of your goals, you can always be successful by learning from your mistakes. Some important and interesting reports about accomplishments and failures are found in a book that I highly recommend, Success by Michael Korda. In this book you are given the guidelines of what it takes to become successful, whether in your personal life or the corporate world.

One important example in Success is the life of Winston Churchill. When he was in school, he had difficulty with English and failed miserably. At times, he was sure he wouldn't graduate. When serving in his country's Army, he was captured by the opposing side, but he escaped. He ran for public office and lost at first, but he tried again and finally became Prime Minister of England. Indeed, he became one of the greatest orators and statesmen of our time. Churchill is an extraordinary example of a man who overcame adversity.

Another exceptional person who achieved success against incredible odds is Bob Wieland. I met Bob in 1979, while I was the Director of the Pritikin Better Health Program. He called me to talk about nutrition and I asked him to attend one of my lectures. After the lecture he came up and introduced himself. I was very impressed with his positive and motivational mental outlook and the sharpness of his mind. He weighed about 242 lbs. at that time, without legs. Bob served our country in Vietnam as a medic, where a bomb mortar exploded and blew off his legs. Only by the grace of God did he survive. Bob wanted to be a seminar speaker, since we were hiring health educators at that time in

1979. Before he started the job, Bob agreed to follow the diet and see what kind of results he could achieve. He followed the plan (personally supervised by me, Nick Delgado) for 10 months. He lost 112 lbs., bringing him to his ideal weight of 130 lbs. (without legs).

I'll never forget the night Bob was scheduled to do a seminar for me in Glendale. The elevators at the hotel had broken down. Bob had a legitimate reason to fold up his wheelchair, call off the seminar and go home - the seminar was to take place on the third floor. Instead he folded up his chair and stacked his seminar supplies: books, projector and screen and proceeded to drag each item up the three flights of stairs, one by one. When people has arrived for the seminar, he was ready. Several people asked him how he got up the stairs without legs in a wheelchair and they were impressed by his "never give up" approach to life.

Bob worked for me until February, 1982 until May, 1986, at which time he embarked on an incredible journey to walk across America on his hands. I worked with Bob again in 1986 by assisting him in the New York City Marathon. Late at night, deep in Harlem, Bob was walking down the dimly lit road. Hungry and tired, but still spirited and determined, we moved slowly down the street. I stopped at a Kentucky Fried Chicken to get us both some food because it was the only place open at that time. What did I get for us? Several large orders of mashed potatoes, corn, rice and beans (this particular location had rice and beans). No chicken, butter or gravy! Bob also ate several apples on his trip. He went on to complete the marathon in just over 90 hours. In the LA Marathon, he broke his previous record. Bob then went on to complete the "Iron Man" Triathalon in Hawaii, a combination of a grueling bike ride (special hand bike for Bob), swimming and running.

Wieland's extraordinary success takes him to colleges, high schools and junior highs to deliver his motivational speeches entitled STRIVE FOR SUCCESS. Bob holds degrees in Physical Education and Recreation. He served six years on the Faculty of the California State University, Los Angeles Physical Education Department, coordinating strength and flexibility programs for athletes. He has appeared on many television and radio broadcasts. He is the only veteran to be named Outstanding Disabled American Veteran in two states (California and Wisconsin). Bob is also a former four-time world champion in the bench press and is an appointee to the President's Council for Fitness and Sports. He will soon be featured in a movie about his life.

Bob doesn't tell you, "I can't follow this diet" or "I don't feel like exercising." You will hear him say how he just enjoyed a new food we recommend and that it's delicious, or "I feel terrific after exercising."

Bob Wieland is an inspiration to all of us. He is my special friend, and when he confided to me his plan to walk across America on his hands, I knew he would succeed. We have maintained our friendship, even as Bob calls me from cities all over the United States. He pours his heart and spirit out to children and adults across this country. Truly a great American and human being, he reminds us of the great potential we all have within us. We all have scars and wounds, whether visible or invisible and Bob is a tribute to just how much man can overcome and accomplish. His attitude is the difference between being successful or not. It is in your mind. You can succeed, so work toward your goals.

We have all experienced failures throughout our lives and sometimes we have felt the last one was the worst that could happen. Unfortunately, something usually comes along to prove us wrong. But, consider the times you failed, but picked yourself up and responded to strengthen yourself. You resolved not to make that mistake again and you realize you have become a better person. We are all built on what is called "good, hard work." From our failures, we become a much stronger individual with stronger character. Don't let failure hold you back; strive for the best. Failures are a key ingredient to developing a better approach to life.

For more information about books, tapes, videos and seminars provided by the Delgado Health Plan, write to P.O. Box:

16787 BEACH BLVD., #202
HUNTINGTON BEACH, CA. 92647

Or come to our office at:

17150 NEWHOPE STREET, SUITE 217
FOUNTAIN VALLEY, CA. 92708

(714) 540-7725

We will send you literature and an order form for you to select products and services to benefit you.

"I need to look great for public appearances, and I enjoy feeling fantastic, having energy, and living according to my values. I must look the picture of health, to serve as a role model for others. A major purpose to my life is to be healthy and vital, and to help as many other people to be as health and vital as they possibly can. The self esteem I have, the respect I gain, the people that I help to reach their goals, makes life all the more enjoyable.

I believe in living a balanced life. It's important to me to maintain high standards of efficiency for myself, my family, and my company. Therefore, a program that takes the minimum amount of time, but yields the greatest results, is of utmost importance to me. When I exercise, I want to get the most out of each session. When I eat, I want to know that beyond the pleasure of eating, I am deriving the maximum benefit of health and vitality from my food choices. I want to utilize my mind for all the wonders the human brain has to offer. Acquiring more knowledge to this end, is one of my driving forces.

I am passionate, and I love living life at the edge. At times, I have to temper this passion, with discipline and delayed gratification, to achieve an even greater result. I am successful, because I am living life according to my values, and not according to other peoples values. I have achieved certain goals that I never thought were possible. Each new day, I look forward to with excitement. Living each day to its fullest. Alive, vital, and full of energy."

- NICK DELGADO

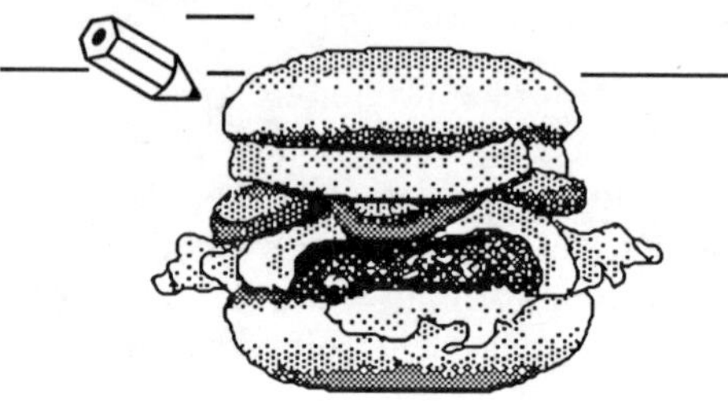

HIGH FAT FAST FOOD

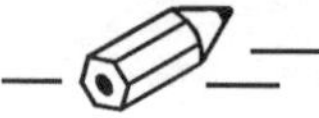

- ✔ Information on cholesterol content of fast foods is not listed. (Remember that foods of animal origin contain cholesterol, so reduce or avoid cheese, meats, creams, etc., when possible).
- ✔ Fast foods are very high in fat, sugar, salt, cholesterol and excess protein. Choose only items recommended.
- ✔ Your total diet should be less than 20% fat. Foods containing over 5 grams of fat should be used in moderation.
- ✔ Fast foods are usually devoid of fiber (except for beans, corn tortillas, vegies & fruit bars and whole wheat sandwiches, which are all good sources of fiber).

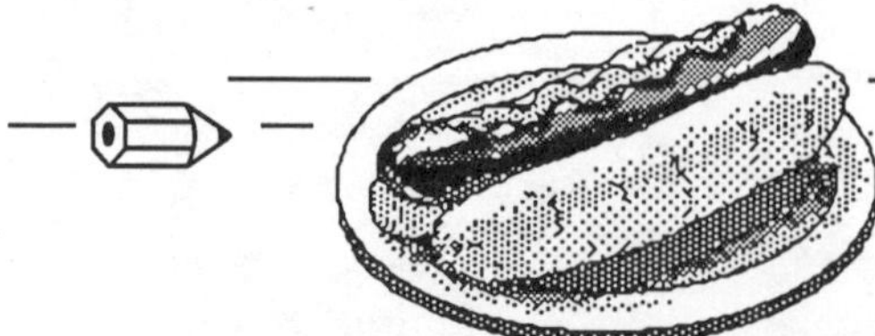

TACO BELL

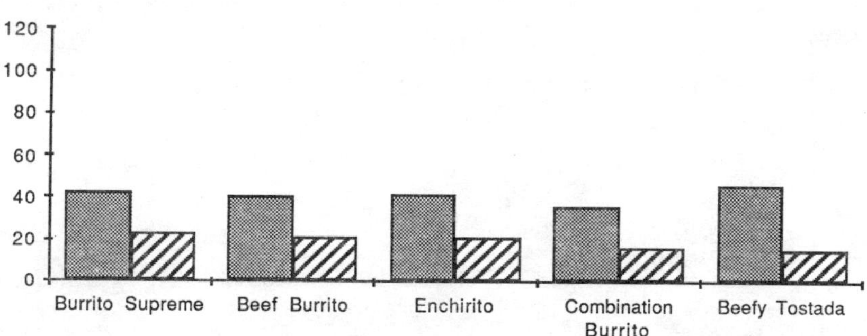

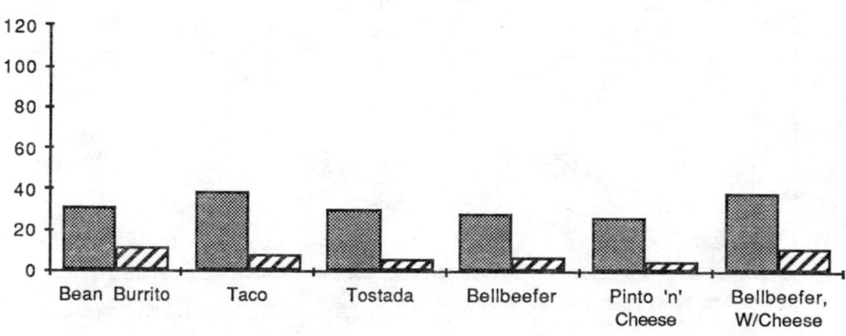

At Taco Bell, order the bean burrito, tostada and Pinto 'n' Cheese without cheese or sour cream and request extra lettuce & tomato with chili salsa (to reduce the fat & cholesterol).

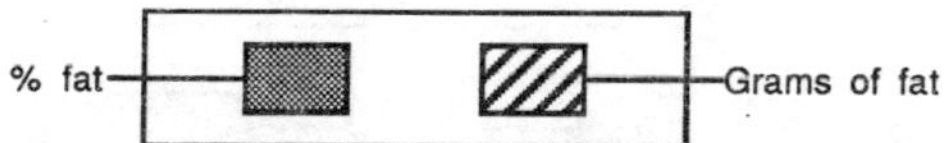

CARL'S JR.

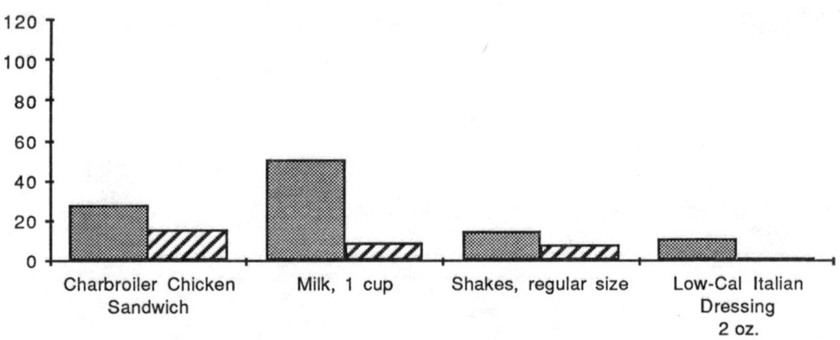

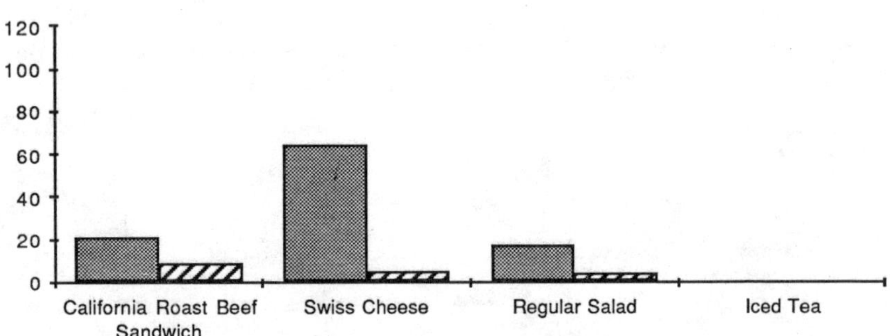

Carl's Jr. has a good salad bar.
You can order the chicken sandwich (pull off the skin) or order the roast beef sandwich without cheese.

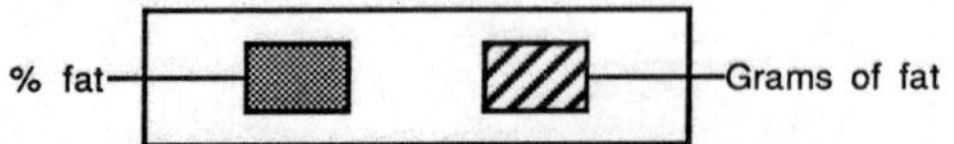

CARL'S JR.

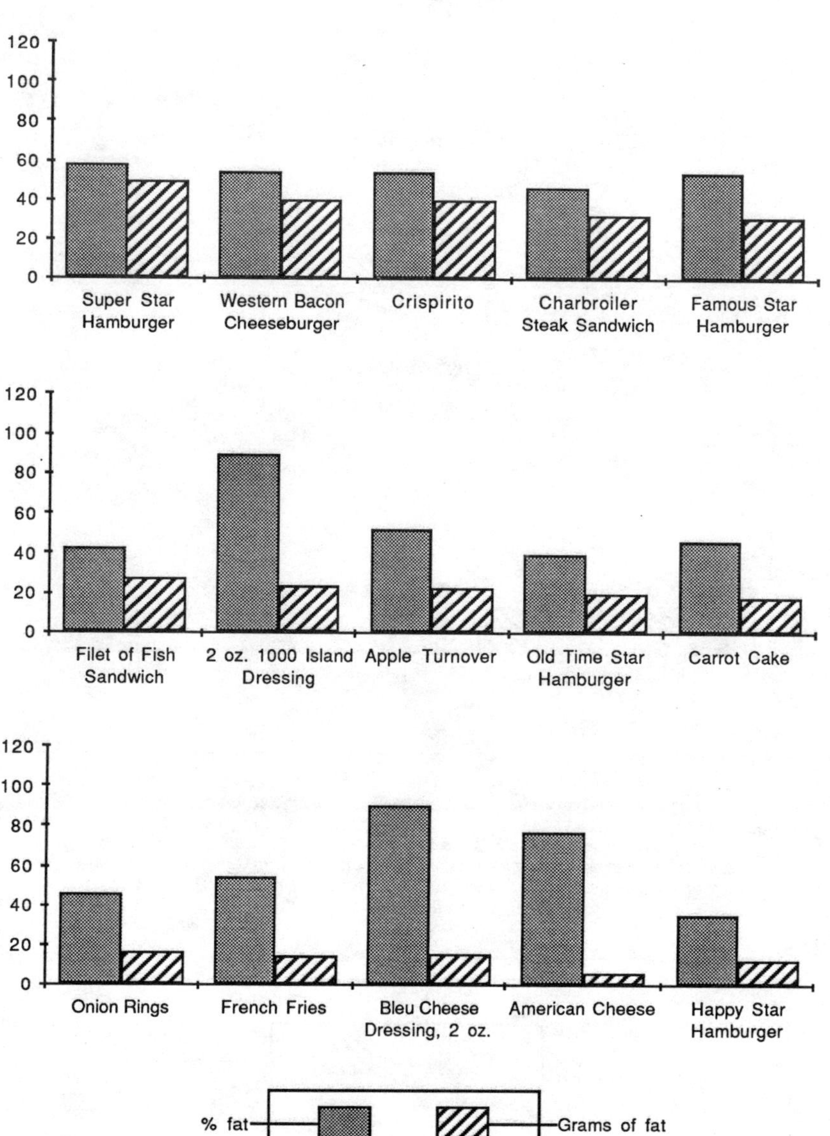
120
100
80
60
40
20
0
Super Star Hamburger
Western Bacon Cheeseburger
Crispirito
Charbroiler Steak Sandwich
Famous Star Hamburger
120
100
80
60
40
20
0
Filet of Fish Sandwich
2 oz. 1000 Island Dressing
Apple Turnover
Old Time Star Hamburger
Carrot Cake
120
100
80
60
40
20
0
Onion Rings
French Fries
Bleu Cheese Dressing, 2 oz.
American Cheese
Happy Star Hamburger
% fat
Grams of fat

PIZZA HUT

1/2 Pizza (10" — 3 slices)
Thin 'n' Crispy

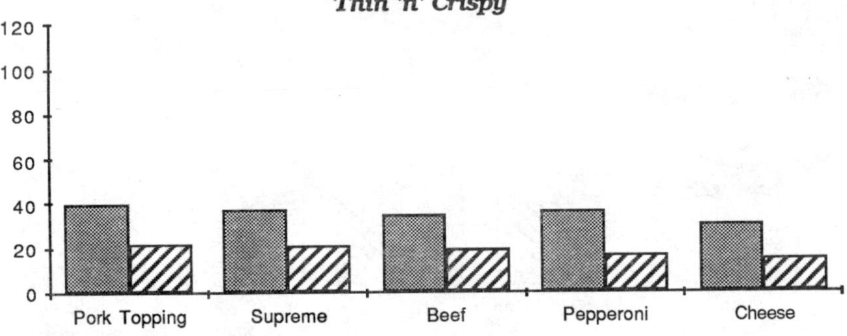

Thick 'n' Chewy

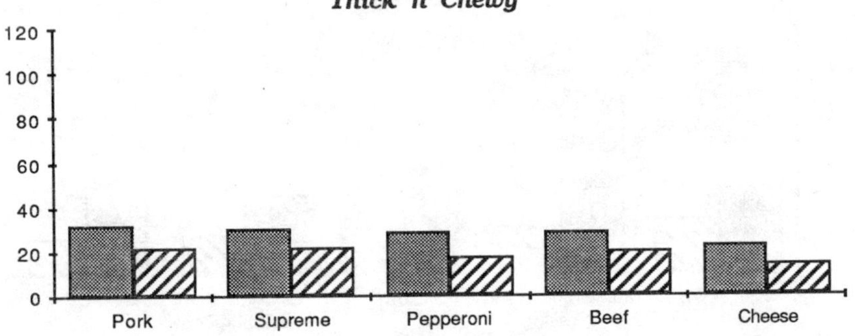

Try to select a pizza parlor that has whole wheat pizza crusts (Wildflour in Redondo Beach . . . see phone book for your area), order your pizza without cheese and ask for extra sauce, tomatoes, mushrooms, onions, bellpeppers, peppers, eggplant, pineapple, etc. You may sprinkle on a small amount of Parmesan cheese (make your own pizza at home with Liteline cheese). Pizza parlors usually have good salad bars.

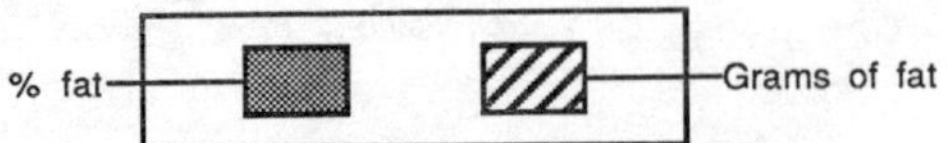

KENTUCKY FRIED CHICKEN

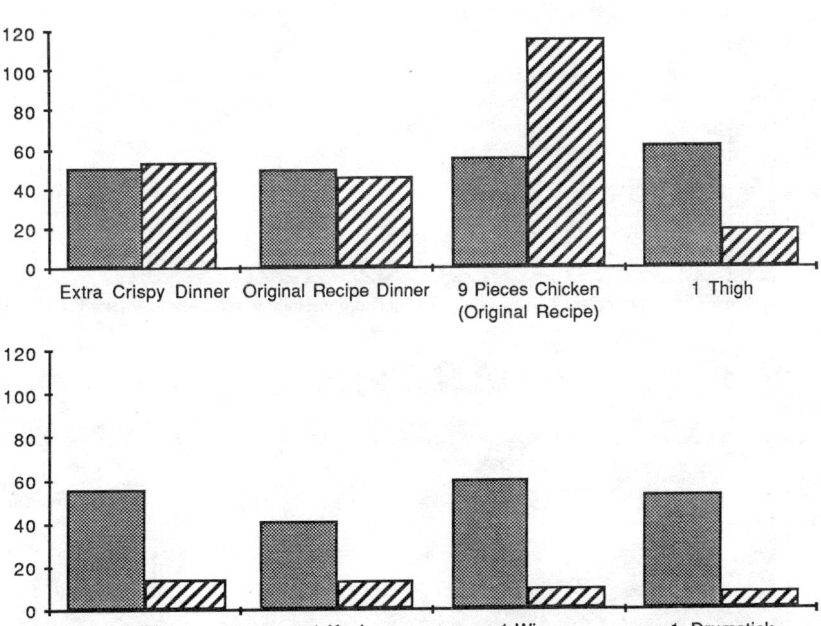

Kentucky Fried Chicken prepares their chicken batter with egg yolks and fries with oil, so be sure to remove the skin to reduce fat and cholesterol. Order mashed potatoes without gravy and corn on the cob (dry off the butter).

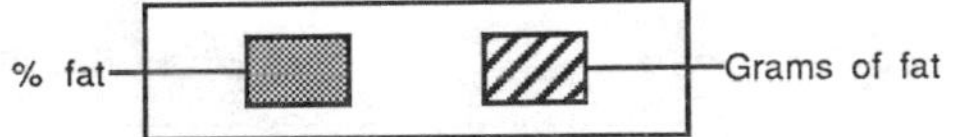

BURGER KING

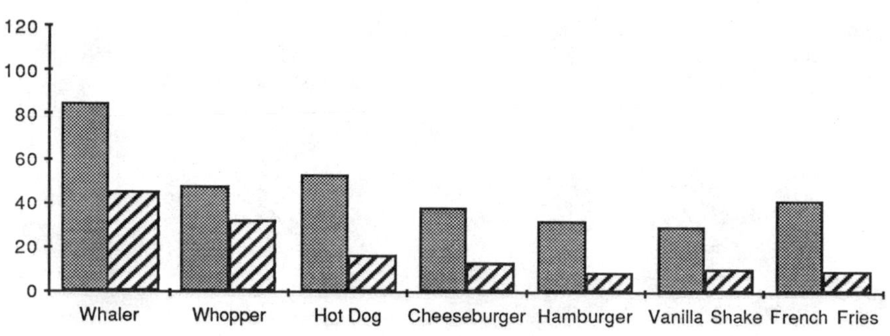

ARBY'S

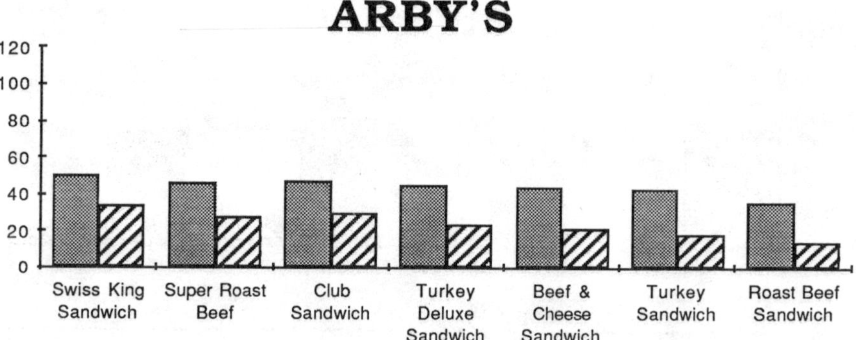

At Arby's, the turkey or roast beef sandwich (without mayonnaise or cheese) could be cut in half, and should be eaten only on rare occasions.

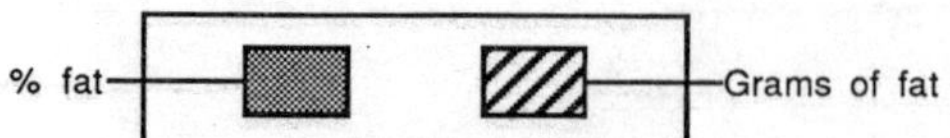

LONG JOHN SILVER'S

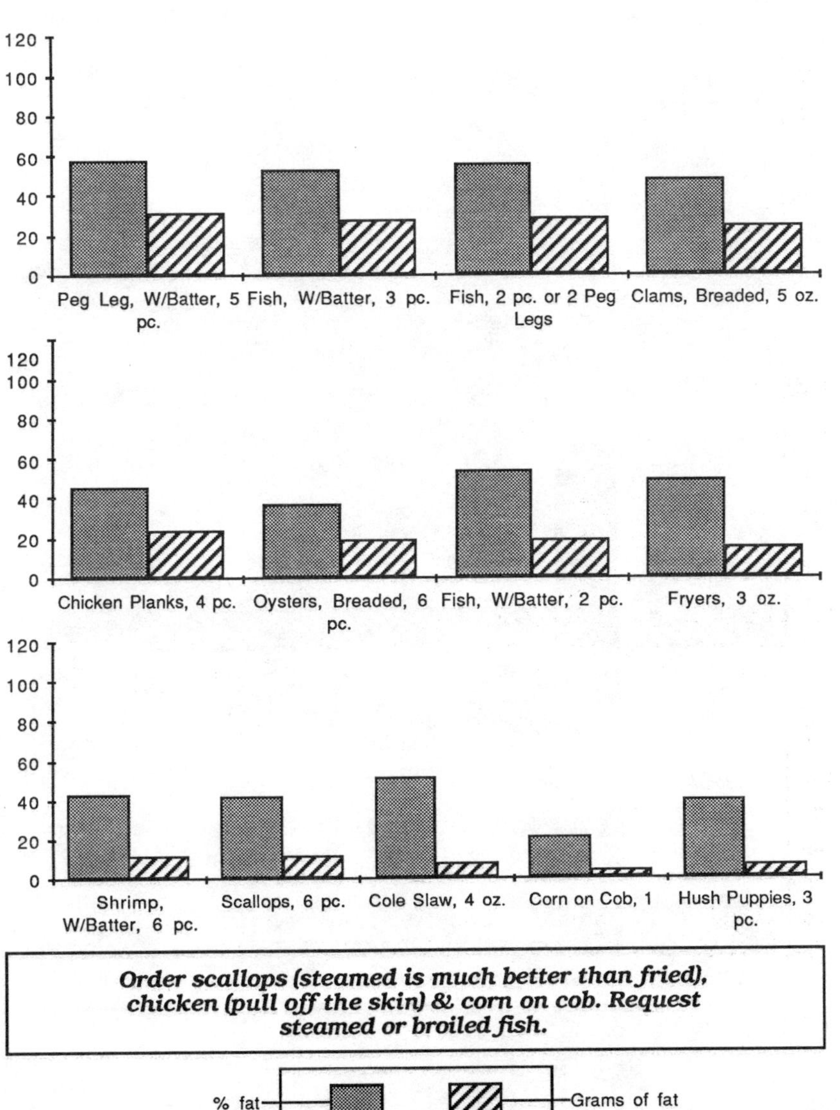

Order scallops (steamed is much better than fried), chicken (pull off the skin) & corn on cob. Request steamed or broiled fish.

McDONALD'S

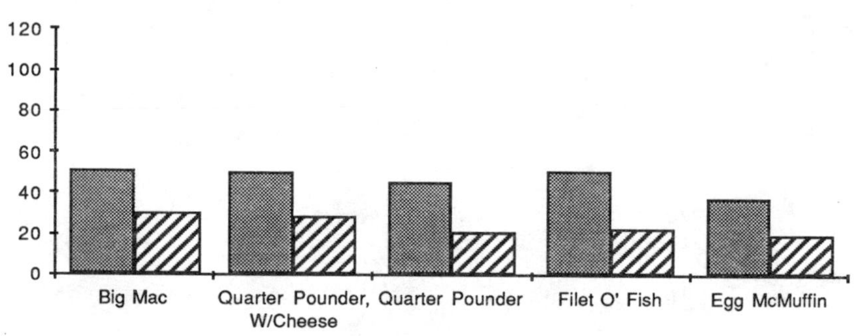

120
100
80
60
40
20
0
Big Mac
Quarter Pounder, W/Cheese
Quarter Pounder
Filet O' Fish
Egg McMuffin

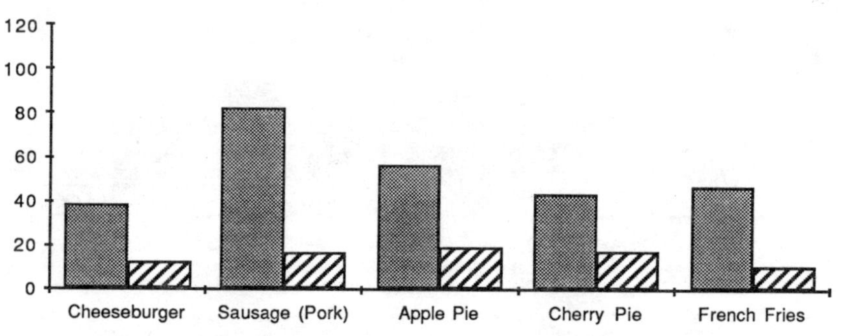

120
100
80
60
40
20
0
Cheeseburger
Sausage (Pork)
Apple Pie
Cherry Pie
French Fries

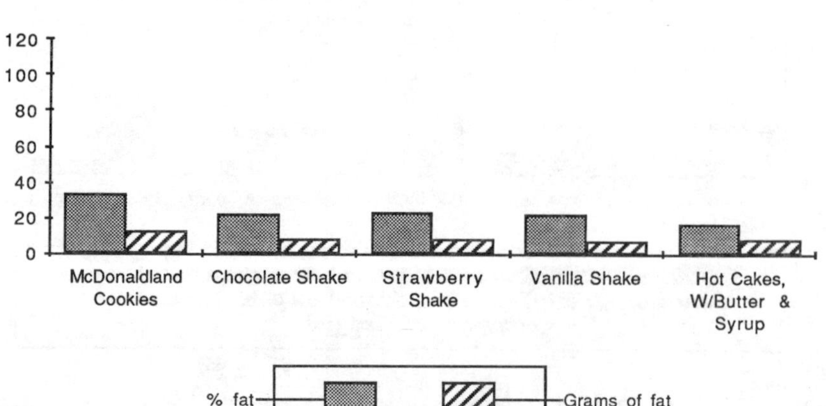

120
100
80
60
40
20
0
McDonaldland Cookies
Chocolate Shake
Strawberry Shake
Vanilla Shake
Hot Cakes, W/Butter & Syrup
% fat
Grams of fat

DAIRY QUEEN

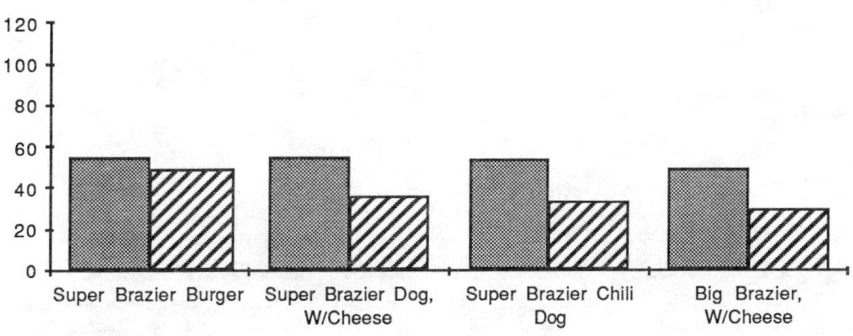

120
100
80
60
40
20
0
Super Brazier Burger
Super Brazier Dog, W/Cheese
Super Brazier Chili Dog
Big Brazier, W/Cheese

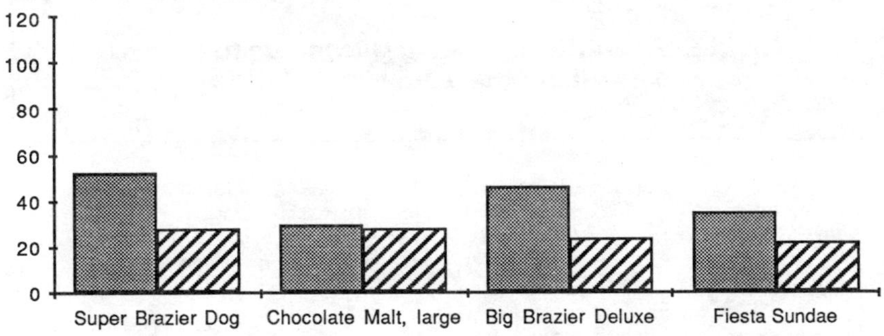

120
100
80
60
40
20
0
Super Brazier Dog
Chocolate Malt, large
Big Brazier Deluxe
Fiesta Sundae

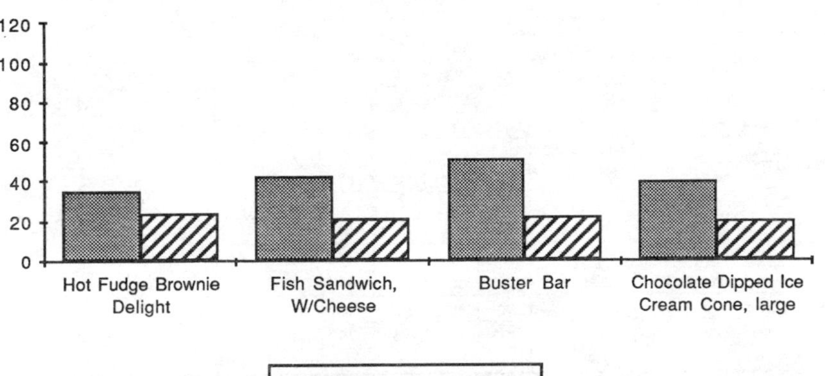

120
100
80
60
40
20
0
Hot Fudge Brownie Delight
Fish Sandwich, W/Cheese
Buster Bar
Chocolate Dipped Ice Cream Cone, large
% fat
Grams of fat

DAIRY QUEEN

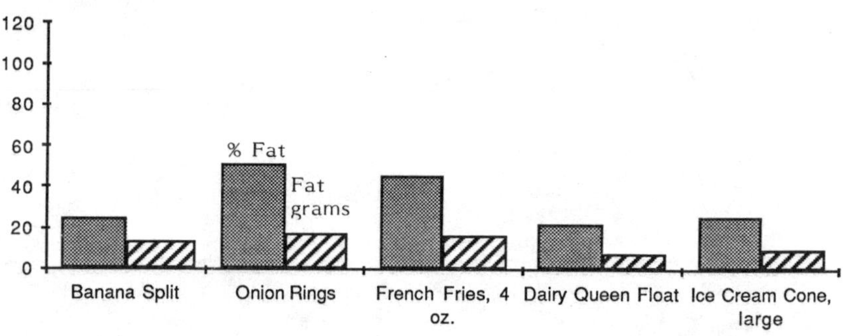

Avoid McDonald's and Dairy Queen due to limited substitution or selection possibilities.

El Pollo Loco promotes their chicken as being a lowfat selection, however notice the excess amount of fat and cholesterol in just two pieces of chicken. A much better choice would be to order the beans, rice, and salsa with corn tortillas to make your own soft tacos. Also order the corn and a salad.

COMBO MEAL: 2 pieces of chicken, salsa, corn, cole slaw and three corn tortillas.	CHICKEN (2 pc.) ♥	SALSA ♥	CORN TORTILLAS ♥	FLOUR TORTILLAS	BEANS	♥ COLE SLAW	CORN ♥	POTATO SALAD ♥	RICE ♥	DOLE WHIP	♥ COMBO
Serving–oz.	4.8*	1.8	3.3	3.3	3.5	2.8	3.3*	4.3	2.5	4.5	16*
Calories	310	10	210	280	110	80	110	140	100	90	720
Protein–g	37	0	6	9	8	2	4	3	3	0	49
Carbohydrates–g	2	1	42	45	17	5	20	15	22	19	70
Fat–g	18	0	2	7	1	6	2	8	1	0	28
% Calories	51	0	8	22	12	67	14	50	9	0	33
Polyunsaturated–g	2	0	1	1	0	3	0	4	na	0	6
Saturated–g	6	0	0	2	1	1	1	1	na	0	8
Cholesterol–mg	80	0	0	0	1	10	0	5	na	0	90
mg/100g	60	0	0	0	1	10	0	5	na	0	20
Sodium–mg	460	90	70	450	450	160	110	500	250	18	890
Potassium–mg	40	25	120	60	25	45	80	70	55	48	310
Fiber–g	0	0	1	1	1	1	1	1	1	0	3

BIBLIOGRAPHY

1. Anderson, James W., M.D. *Diabetes - A practical new guide to healthy living*. New York, New York: Arco Publishing, Inc., 1981.
2. Bailey, Covert. *The Fit-or-Fat Target Diet*. Boston, Massachusetts: Houghton Mifflin Company, 1984.
3. Bennett, Cleaves M., M.D. *In 12 weeks you can control your high blood pressure without drugs*. Garden City, New York: Doubleday & Company, Inc., 1984.
4. Bronfen, Nan. *Nutrition for a Better Life*. Santa Barbara, California: Capra Press, 1980.
5. Burkitt, Denis, M.D., F.R.C.S., F.R.S. *Eat right - to stay healthy and enjoy life more*. New York, New York: Arco Publishing, 1979.
6. Dunne, Lavon J. *Nutrition Almanac*. New York, New York: McGraw Hill Publishing Company, 1990.
7. Guyton, Arthur C., M.D. *Textbook of Medical Physiology*. Philadelphia, Pennsylvania: W.B. Sanders Company, 1976.
8. Klaper, Michael, M.D. *Pregnancy, Children and the Vegan Diet*. Umatilla, Florida: Gentle World Inc., 1987.
9. Langley, Gill, M.A., Ph.D. *Vegan Nutrition*. Oxford, England: The Vegan Society Ltd., 1988.
10. Leonard, Jon N., and J.L. Hofer and Nathan Pritikin. *Live Longer Now*.
11. McDougall, John A., M.D. *McDougall's Medicine*. Piscataway, New Jersey: New Century Publishers, Inc., 1985.
12. McDougall, John A., M.D., and Mary A. McDougall. *The McDougall Plan*. Piscataway, New Jersey: New Century Publishers, Inc., 1983.
13. Pritikin, Nathan. *The Pritikin Permanent Weight Loss Manual*. New York, New York: Grosset and Dunlap, 1981.
14. Pritikin, Nathan. *The Pritikin Program for Diet and Exercise*. New York, New York: Grosset and Dunlap, 1979.
15. Robbins, John. *Diet for a New America*. Walpole, New Hampshire: Stillpoint Publishing, 1987.
16. Sattilaro, Anthony J., M.D. *Recalled for Life*. New York, New York: Avon Books, 1982.

BIBLIOGRAPHY

17. Swank, Roy Haver, M.D., and Barbara Brewer Dugan. *The Multiple Sclerosis Diet Book*. New York, New York: Doubleday, 1977.
18. Webb, Densie, Ph.D., R.D. *The Complete "Lite" Foods Calorie, Fat, Cholesterol and Sodium Counter*. New York, New York: Bantam Books, 1990.
19. Whitaker, Julian M., M.D. *Reversing Diabetes*. New York, New York: Warner Books, Inc., 1987.
20. Whitaker, Julian M., M.D. *Reversing Heart Disease*. New York, New York: Warner Books, Inc., 1985.

ABOUT THE AUTHOR

More than 14 years ago, Nick Delgado was 50 lbs. overweight, had high blood pressure and considered clinically obese. In his search for a solution to his own health problems, he discovered the best approach was a unique nutrition and exercise program. Nick lost 50 lbs. of unwanted fat and reduced his blood pressure and cholesterol to safe levels permanently.

Nick was awarded a full State and University scholastic scholarship to the University of Southern California, where he received a B.A. in Psychology in 1977. He completed six months of Master's work in Physical Therapy at USC's Rancho Los Amigos Hospital in 1977. He went to Loma Linda University in 1982, where he was accepted into their Health Science program as a Masters and Doctoral candidate. Nick worked with the Nathan Pritikin Longevity Center, Santa Monica, California presenting education conferences and scientific studies from 1979-1981. Since then, Nick has professionally conducted 3,200 seminars, workshops and conventions form 1979-1991. Topics have included stress and weight reduction, nutrition, exercise, prevention of disease, quality health and happiness. Nick's goal is to establish health education programs nationally and internationally and in the process help everyone become as healthy and happy as they can.

THE DELGADO HEALTH PLAN
HAS CHANGED THE LIVES OF OUR PARTICIPANTS!

Mr. AND MRS. JOHN KENT, *"John's cholesterol level is down...his blood pressure went to normal...and we both lost weight. His heart specialist is impressed - saying it's the most dramatic improvement he's seen."*

WALT HERD, *"I have a great feeling of excitement and accomplishment since starting the program. I started your program right after the results of my blood test came in. The results revealed a cholesterol level of 242, exactly 100 points higher than it should be for my age. This frightened me into action because my father had just had a seven-way - yes, 7-way - bypass operation and in no way was I interested in being in that position in my future. So, in earnest I followed your program and in seven weeks my cholesterol was reduced to 144. AND I FEEL GREAT ABOUT IT!"*

HAROLD E. KIMZEY, *"Some of the problems I was trying to control or eliminate will be familiar to many. Now in my early 60's, I was 60 to 70 pounds overweight and a borderline diabetic. I had high blood pressure, high triglycerides and suffered from irregularity of my bowels. In the short time that I've been with Delgado Medical, I've found that my blood pressure is returning to normal, my triglycerides are coming down, I am no longer diabetic, I have regular bowel movements and I've lost 20 pounds. Also, my energy level has increased and I'm aware of a keener sense of well being. Who can beat that?"*

RICHARD SHUTA, *"The Delgado Health Plan immmediately brought my blood pressure down within a matter of a few weeks. I feel great. I'm going to be around as a healthy individual, not someone who is crippled up with problems or dependent on medication."*

THERESA GESKE, *"When I started the Plan, the first thing I noticed I started feeling less tired. I could think clearer, too. In a period of about three to four weeks, I could really see changes starting to take place. The Plan did wonders for me. It made me feel better, much more energetic."*